Milks Alive

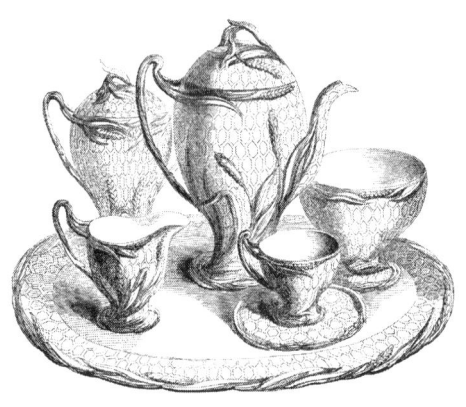

RITA RIVERA

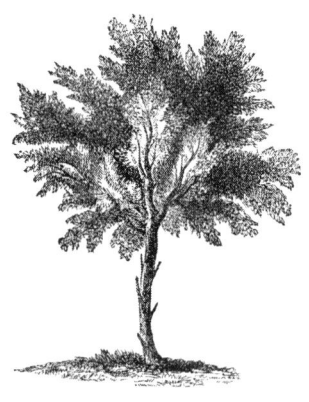

*This book is dedicated to "Pachamama,"
our beautiful, abundant Mother Earth.*

*If we listen, she will teach us,
the heart of being and the art of living.*

*Each day is a practice in love,
harmony and deep reverence
for each other,
the precious animals,
the land,
the waters
and
the air that sustains us...*

Milks Alive

Santa Cruz, California
United States of America
rita@milksalive.com
www.milksalive.com

©2013 Rita Rivera. All rights reserved. Printed in the United States of America. Except as permitted under the United States Copyright Act of 1976, no part of this publication may be reproduced, distributed in any form or by any means, or entered in a database or retrieval system without the prior written consent of the Author.

Book Design: Diane Rigoli, RigoliCreative.com
Cover Photo Shot by: Betty Ann Rosa-Galderisi
www.beauricua.com/beautyblog
Illustrations: Courtesy FCIT, Shutterstock

10 9 8 7 6 5 4 3 2 1

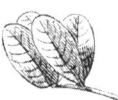 # Contents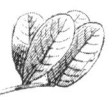

Introduction 1
My Story 3
Acknowledgments 5
Basic Information 7
Ingredient List 9
Getting Started 15
Equipment 15
Soaking, Blending & Straining 16
To Blanche or Not to Blanche 18
Leftover Pulp 19
Storage & Shelf Life 19

NUTS

ALMONDS 21
   Simple Unsweetened Almond Milk 22
   Almond Milk Ratios 23
   Almond Milk from Almond Butter 26
   Date Almond Milk 28
   Honey Almond Milk 29
   Apple Almond Milk 29
   Apple Lime Almond Milk 30
   Pear & Candied Ginger Almond Milk 30
   Cranberry Almond Milk 31
   Sweet & Sour Gooseberry Almond Milk 31
   Maple Orange Almond Milk 32
   Raisin Cinnamon Almond Milk 32
   Banana Fig Almond Smoothie 32
   Pineapple Ginger Almond Milk 33
   Pineapple Orange Apricot Almond Milk . . . 33
   Goji Berry Pomegranate Honey Almond Milk . . . 34
   Prune Almond Milk 34
   Prune & Candied Ginger Almond Milk 35
   Prune Banana Ginger Almond Smoothie . . . 35

    Carrot Almond Milk 35
    Carrot Pineapple Almond Milk 36
    Kale Apple Almond Milk 36
    Kale Apple & Fresh Ginger Almond Milk 37
    Kale Celery Apple Almond Milk. 37
    Kale Pear Banana & Seed Mix Almond Smoothie . . 38
    Kale Apple Banana Hemp & Almond Smoothie . . 38
    Wheatgrass Kale Apple Almond Milk 39
    Wheatgrass Kale Apple Lime Almond Milk 40
    Wheatgrass Kale Orange Almond Milk. 40
    Wheatgrass Kale Celery Apple Almond Milk. . . 41
    Wheatgrass Kale Celery Lemon Apple &
        Ginger Almond Milk 42

VANILLA 43
    Making Fresh Vanilla Liquid 44
    Vanilla Almond Milk 45
    Chocolate Almond Milk 46
    Hot Chocolate Almond Milk 46
    Chocolate Peppermint Almond Milk 47
    Mesquite Chocolate Malt Almond Milk 47
    Carob Almond Milk 47
    Carob Malted Almond Milk 48
    Carob Malted Almond Smoothie 48
    Orange Blossom Almond Milk 49

COCONUTS 51
    Opening A Young Thai Coconut 53
    Fresh Coconut Milk 54
    Almond Coconut Milk 55
    Coco Loco 55
    Coco Loco Supreme 55
    Pina Colada 56
    Pineapple Banana Colada Smoothie. 56
    Pineapple Banana Ginger Colada Smoothie . . . 56
    Coconut Milk from Shredded Dried Coconut . . . 57

CASHEWS 59
- Simple Cashew Milk. 60
- Sweet Cashew Milk. 61
- Creamy Cashew Coconut Milk. 61
- Cashew Almond Date Milk 61
- Vegan Egg Nog. 62
- Cashew Hemp Milk. 62
- Cashew Hemp Chocolate Milk. 63
- Cashew Hemp Orange Vanilla Milk. 63
- Cashew Hemp Orange Vanilla Banana Smoothie. . 63
- Lavender Honey Cashew Milk 64
- Lavender Honey Simple Syrup 64
- Lavender Honey & Ginger Sparkling Cashew Milk . 65
- Cashew Pomegranate Orange Milk. 65

BRAZIL NUTS 67
- Simple Brazil Nut Milk. 68
- Creamy Brazil Nut Milk 68
- Creamy Brazil Praline Smoothie 69
- Brazil Almond Milk 69
- Brazil Almond Goji Berry Milk 69
- Brazil Almond Chocolate Mint Milk. 70
- Peach Banana Brazil Nut Smoothie 70
- Raspberry Coconut Anise Brazil Nut Smoothie . . 70

WALNUTS 71
- Simple Walnut Milk. 72
- Walnut Date Milk. 73
- Creamy Walnut Coconut Milk 73
- Creamy Walnut Coconut Cinnamon & Honey Milk. 74
- Walnut Almond Milk. 74
- Walnut Almond Raisin Milk 74
- Walnut Almond Fall Smoothie 75
- Walnut Almond Anise Milk 75
- Walnut Almond Anise Orange Milk 75
- Walnut Oat Milk 76
- Walnut Oat Raisin Milk. 76

  Walnut Oat Raisin Banana Smoothie 76
  Walnut Pear Milk 77
  Walnut Pear Pomegranate Milk 77
  Walnut Pear Pomegranate Milk & Greens 77

HAZELNUTS 79
  Simple Hazelnut Milk 80
  Creamy Hazelnut Milk 81
  Sweetened Hazelnut Milk. 81
  Chocolate Hazelnut Milk 82
  Hot Chocolate Hazelnut Milk 82
  Hazelnut Orange Date Milk 82
  Hazelnut Orange Raspberry Smoothie 82
  Hazelnut Banana Cinnamon Smoothie 83
  Hazel Brazil Nut Milk 83
  Hazel Brazil Nut Chocolate Milk 83
  Hazel Brazil Nut Decadence 84

PEANUTS 85
  Simple Peanut Milk 86
  Sweetened Peanut Milk 87
  Peanut Grape Milk 87
  Peanut Banana Honey Smoothie 87
  Peanut Chocolate Milk 88
  Peanut Chocolate Malt Banana Smoothie 88
  Peanut Sesame Milk 88
  Peanut Sesame Chocolate Banana Smoothie . . . 88

MACADAMIA NUTS 89
  Simple Macadamia Nut Milk 90
  Sweetened Macadamia Nut Milk 90
  Macadamia Coconut Milk. 91
  Macadamia Banana Coconut Smoothie 91

COFFEE & NUT MILK 93
    Frothing Nut Milk. 94
    Almond Milk for Coffee & Lattes 94
    Hazelnut Milk for Coffee & Lattes 94
    Iced Coffee 95
    Coffee Substitutes. 96

TEAS & NUT MILK 97
    Chai Tea & Almond Milk 99
    Bengal Spice Tea & Almond Milk 99
    Rooibos Tea & Almond Milk. 100
    Rooibos Tea & Coconut Milk 100
    Matcha Green Tea & Almond Milk 101
    Matcha Green Tea with Hemp & Banana. 101

SODA FOUNTAIN CREAMS WITH ALMOND MILK . . . 103
    Chocolate Soda Fountain Cream 104
    Grape Soda Fountain Cream. 104
    Orange Soda Fountain Cream 105

NUT MILKSHAKES 105

🌰 SEEDS 🌰

HEMP SEEDS 107
    Simple Hemp Milk 108
    Sweetened Hemp Milk 109
    Vanilla Hemp Milk 109
    Hemp Milk with Coconut Water 110
    Hemp Almond Milk with Coconut Water & Chia . 110
    Hemp Cashew Milk 110
    Hemp Cashew Orange Date Milk. 111
    Hemp Persimmon Smoothie 111
    Hemp Persimmon Honey Cinnamon Smoothie . . 111
    Hemp Pomegranate Coconut Banana Smoothie . . 112

SUNFLOWER SEEDS 113
   Simple Sunflower Milk 115
   Creamy Sunflower Milk 115
   Sweetened Sunflower Milk 115
   Toffee Sunflower Milk 116
   Sunflower Banana Milk. 116
   Sunflower Persimmon Cranberry Smoothie. . . . 117
   Sunflower Pecan Vanilla Milk 117
   Sunflower Pecan Vanilla Smoothie 118
   Sunflower Hemp Coconut Grape Milk 118

PUMPKIN SEEDS 119
   Simple Pumpkin Seed Milk 120
   Creamy Pumpkin Seed Milk 121
   Sweetened Pumpkin Seed Milk. 121
   Pumpkin Seed Wheatgrass Milk 121
   Creamy Pumpkin Seed Coconut Milk 122

CHIA SEEDS 123
   Chia Seeds with Nut or Seed Milk 124
   Chia Seed Smoothies. 124
   Chia Seed Iced Tea 125

OTHER SEEDS & NUTS 127
   Pecans 128
   Pistachios 130
   Pine Nuts 131
   Sesame Seeds 132
   Flax Seeds 134

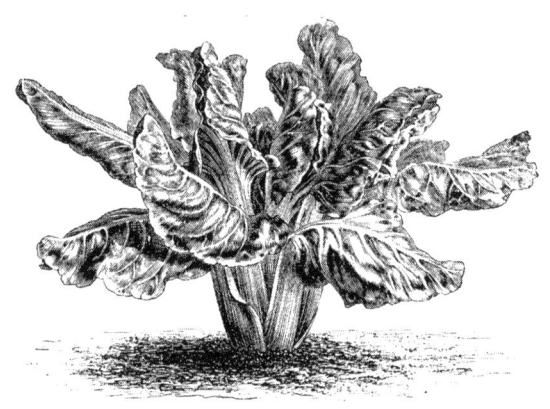

Introduction

We live in a fast-paced and changing world, a world where we are continually challenged to create balance in our lives and to make educated choices about our lifestyles. Without thoughtful and intentional decisions, the health and balance of both our bodies and our planet pay the price.

Needless to say, the price has been high; obesity, diabetes, cancers and heart disease are at epidemic proportions. The rise of industrialized farming and the corporatization of food have forced many family farms out of business. Factory-farmed animals suffer greatly, never seeing the light of day or a green pasture. Quantity is replacing quality, and the sustainable care of our land is overshadowed and driven by profits.

At the *heart* of the matter, our individual choices and decisions are affecting our health, the health of our families and the balance of our planet.

We are surrounded by extraordinary choices in food and beverages. From super grocery stores to kiosks, from high-end gourmet restaurants to fast food, from food shows on television and endless food commercials, we are inundated with tastes and flavors from near and far.

A strong movement is emerging! More and more people are embracing slow food and local, organic and urban gardening. Plant-based foods that are delicious, nutritious, colorful and fresh are inspiring many to explore vegetarian, vegan and raw food diets; and it's changing their bodies, their health, and their philosophies about living and consuming in our modern world.

Parents know that kids especially require high-quality foods to provide the necessary nutrition for them to achieve their peak potential. My "Green Milk Blends," in the presence of kids, becomes the "Green Monster Smoothie." Little do they know that they are drinking their greens! It's a delight to see little green mustaches on smiley faces holding out glasses for more.

You will find many "kid friendly" recipes in my book. For high quality fats, you can add a slice of avocado for creaminess. Check out the Vegan Nog recipe! Bananas will add both sweetness and creaminess, and using a fruit juice base adds the right touch of sweetness to balance the greens. Check out the kale and wheatgrass recipes!

When we make these fresh nut and seed milks at home, we know exactly what we are consuming as we prepare quality, nutrient-rich beverages with great taste that will feed and fuel happy, healthy, vital bodies.

This book is devoted to those who are sensitive to dairy, lactose intolerant or simply interested in making healthy choices. I am thrilled and delighted to share my nut and seed milk recipes with you and to encourage the use of plant-based milks as an alternative or as an adjunct to dairy products.

So many flavors to explore...

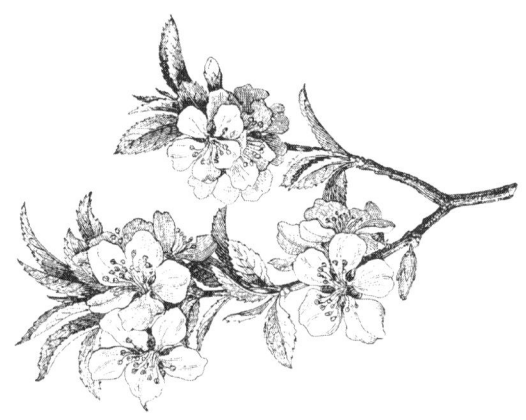

My Story

Many years ago I was visiting a friend on the Big Sur coast in northern California who was just getting into a diet of raw, vegan foods. I could not imagine adopting such a diet; a piece of raw broccoli on a plate was not appetizing! And the thought of drinking milk made from nuts sounded crazy to me!

Little did I know that this weekend would change the course of my health and my life. What great fortune to be introduced to freshly made almond milk and the beauty of raw food preparation. That particular beautiful, warm weekend we spent many hours in the kitchen experimenting with making milks from different nuts with a variety of flavorings and sweeteners—silky, creamy, delicious elixirs!

With an expansive view of the Pacific ocean from the kitchen window, it was a magical weekend and I was excited to learn about this new way of experiencing food.

A few days after returning home, I literally began to crave the freshly made almond milk. The craving was so strong that I continued to make the milks and to research the nutrient value of nuts, as it became obvious that my body wanted more of this type of food.

Frustratingly, for most of my adult life, I accepted the fact that I had allergies and sinus problems. It never occurred to me that my allergy symptons were related to the foods that I was eating. I began to understand that although I was not lactose intolerant, I did have an acute sensitivity to dairy and soy products. My biggest surprise was when I took dairy and soy out of my diet. Within a week my struggle with "allergies" went away and my digestive issues as well!

MILKS ALIVE IS BORN
After several years of preparing fresh nut and seed milks and being at a transitional point in my life, I started Milks Alive and sold fresh-pressed almond milk blends at local farmers markets in Santa Cruz and Monterey counties in California. In a short amount of time, we built a strong following and our rapid growth had us poised to expand into a wholesale line for several northern California retail stores.

Before I made my final decision and committments to move forward with the growth of my company, I took some time to weigh out my options and gave myself the gift of quiet, comtemplative time. I came to the conclusion that it was best for me to step back and take time to write my first recipe book and and re-vision the path for Milks Alive.

It is my hope that the power packed plant-based milk recipes that you will find in my book will impact your health and energy as it did mine!

Enjoy!
Rita

Visit our website:
www.MilksAlive.com

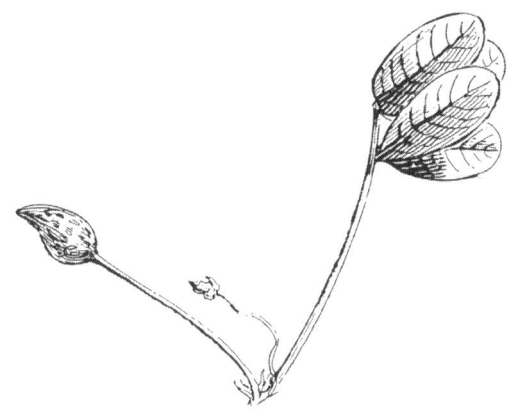

Acknowledgments

Special thanks to those who have supported me on this journey in bringing this book to you: Shana, Peter & Kyra Phelan, Laurie & Michael Groves, Nanette Ruggiero, Richie & Betty Galderisi, Nancy Lowe, Drew Goodwin, Anthony Casolino, Darcy Elman, Irene Stephens & Cooper Gallegos, Sharon Mazer, Laurie Rubin, Lisa Carter, Dent de Lion Du Midi, Deborah Regina, Ronald Regina, Gail Moore, Jennifer Torborg, Joy Binah, Helen Jones, Carol Hwang Fields, Christine Miller, Cindie Ambar, Leslie Arutunian, Meagan Hawk, Zeina Smidi, Tom Quinn, Karen Mehringer, Allyson Rampage, Ellen Bucci.

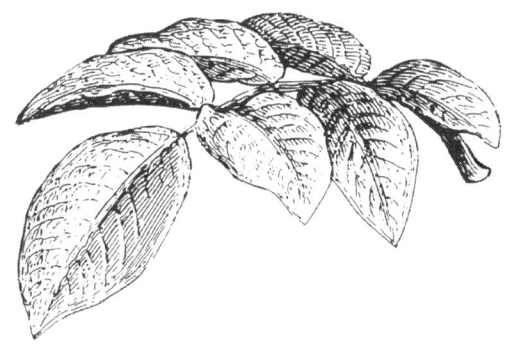

Basic Information

Go organic.
Purchase non-GMO foods.
Vary nuts and seeds in your diet.
Celebrate greens in your daily food choices.
Incorporate low gyclemic sweeteners.
Use filtered water.

- My recipes are designed to prepare milk with a smooth and silky texture! This requires straining after blending, using a quality nut mik bag or cheese cloth.

- All recipes call for nuts and seeds in their raw state, unsalted and unprocessed. Soaking times of nuts and seeds will vary; not all nuts and seeds require soaking. Recipe measurements call for dry nuts or seeds before they are soaked.

- Smoothies and milkshakes have a thicker consistency and denser texture.

- Many of these recipes can be "tweaked" to satisfy your taste profile, by adding a little more of this or a little less of that.

- Single portion recipes can be doubled and quart recipes can be cut into quarters or in half, depending on your needs.

THE GLYCEMIC INDEX AND SUGARS

The "Glycemic Index" is a good thing to familiarize yourself with when considering your sugar intake and choices in sweeteners.

The Glycemic Index measures the rate of speed that sugars and carbohydrates have on blood sugar levels. Foods that rapidly release glucose into the blood are rated high on the glycemic index. Foods that slowly release glucose are low on the glycemic index. Mixing high and low GI foods can result in a moderate glucose release.

Think of it like this: there are "fast" sugars and "slow" sugars. Slow sugars do not spike glucose levels, whereas fast sugars are immediately released into the bloodstream, causing your blood glucose levels to rise. The rise in blood glucose stimulates an insulin response by the pancreas to stabilize blood sugar. Excess carbohydrates and "fast" sugars can cause serious health issues such as weight gain, high cholesterol, cardiovascular disease, bowel disorders, high blood pressure and diabetes.

I use a variety of sweeteners in my recipes that are predominately low on the GI scale, along with simple milk recipes that do not add sweeteners.

Your intuition, creativity and joy are the best assets to bring into the kitchen.

Have fun!

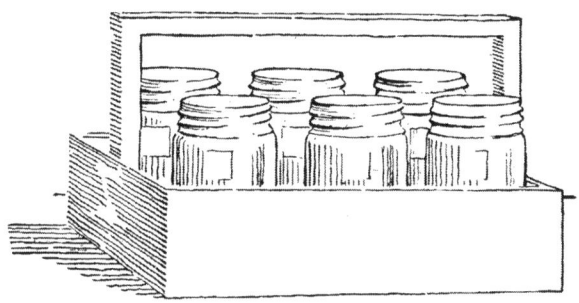

Ingredient List

You may or may not be familiar with some ingredients that I use in my recipes. You can find most of them at your local health food store, or you can visit our website for links on where to purchase them.

AGAVE
Agave plants thrive in the volcanic soils of southern Mexico with over 100 species that come in many sizes and colors.

The agave plant, most well known for producing tequila, also produces a sap that is processed and used as a sweetener. The heart of the plant is pressed, filtered and heated to extract the agave juice to break down the carbohydrates into sugar.

Although widely accepted in the mainstream market, there has been some controversy regarding the fructose content, which varies from different companies. Always purchase organic and use sparingly, or substitute another sweetener of choice.

CAROB
The carob tree is characteristic of the Mediterranean region and is found all over the Middle East. The carob tree produces a pod that contains the carob bean, also known as locust bean.

The carob beans are dried and then made into a powder. Carob powder can be found raw or roasted and has a wonderful subtle flavor that resembles chocolate and is often used as a substitute for chocolate.

The carob bean provides some emulsifying and thickening properties, however I use it solely for its delicious flavor!

CACAO / CHOCOLATE POWDER
The "chocolate tree" or cacao tree, indigenous to Central and South America is now grown in tropical climates worldwide. Our beloved chocolate is made from the cacao beans of the cacao tree.

According to FDA guidelines, cocoa powder and cacao powder are simply different terms for the same powder and are nearly interchangeable; however, "cacao powder" specifically refers to low heat, unsweetened powder. Cocoa powder may be processed with high heat and or chemicals and may still contain a small amount of cocoa butter.

CHICORY
Chicory contains a compound called fructo-oligosaccharides or more commonly know as FOS. The FOS compound found naturally in chicory is inulin, which is a carbohydrate fiber. FOS and inulin have gained attention for their health promoting benefits as prebiotics. Prebiotics are substances that are able to reach the colon to be utilized by the beneficial intestinal flora and support probiotics that maintain our intestinal health.

Chicory in the right quantity will add a subtle sweetness and enhance texture.

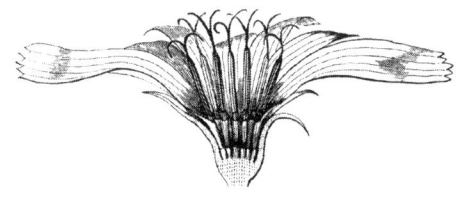

COCONUT PALM SUGAR

Coconut palm sugar is made from a nutrient rich sap that is tapped from the coconut blossoms of the coconut palm tree. This sap is low glycemic, containing amino acids, minerals, vitamin C, B vitamins and it resembles brown sugar.

GOJI BERRY, OR WOLFBERRY

Goji berries are rich in antioxidants and have been used by herbalists for thousands of years in China, Tibet and India.

When dried, the goji berry has a beautiful red-orange color and looks like a raisin. It and can be found in temperate and subtropical regions in China, Mongolia and Tibet.

LECITHIN

Lecithin is a lipid, composed of choline and inositol, and is found in all living cells as a major component of cell membranes.

Lecithin acts an emulsifier, keeping the ingredients mixed together, preventing separation. For nutritional reasons and for less separation in your milks, lecithin can be added to most recipes.

I recommend the powdered form and always certified organic, non-GMO!

MACA

Maca is a cruciferous root vegetable that resembles a turnip or a large radish and grows in extreme conditions at very high altitudes in Peru and Ecuador.

Native cultures have used maca for thousands of years and maca is known for its ability to increase energy and stamina and to stimulate and balance hormonal activity in both men and women.

Maca has a very rich nutrient profile with numerous phytochemicals, amino acids, beneficial fatty acids and vitamins.

MESQUITE

The mesquite tree is found around the world and is native to deserts. This heat and drought tolerant tree produces a malty, subtle, caramel-flavor bean pod, which is ground into a meal.

Mesquite is a slow-acting carbohydrate and helps balance and control blood sugar absorption. Mesquite is mineral-rich, including trace minerals and approximately 15% protein.

STEVIA

Stevia is part of the sunflower family, native to subtropical and tropical regions, and is widely grown for its sweet leaves. Try taking a bite from the leaf of a stevia plant—you can taste the sweetness!

Stevia extracts have up to 300 times the sweetness of sugar and have a low effect on blood glucose levels.

The one drawback to using stevia is often a bitter aftertaste. If you are unfamiliar with stevia, begin with very small amounts.

TOCOTRIENOLS (TOCOS)

Stabilized rice tocotrienols, also called rice solubles, have a light, fluffy texture and are the nutritional powerhouse of the rice grain. The rice grain provides the most important nutrients for the sprouting rice plant and the bran contains proteins, minerals, vitamins and healthy fats.

Tocos, high in vitamin E, are a slightly sweet tasting supplement that provide the natural mix of tocopherols and tocotrienols.

They easily dissolve in our milk blends and add both texture and a subtle sweetness.

XYLITOL

Xylitol is a naturally occurring carbohydrate found widely in fruits and vegetables and is used as a sweetener. For commercial purpose, xylitol is made from Birch tree bark or from corn husks.

Xylitol tastes and looks like sugar, however it has 40% fewer calories and does not raise insulin or affect blood sugar levels.

If you purchase xylitol produced from corn, purchase organic xylitol.

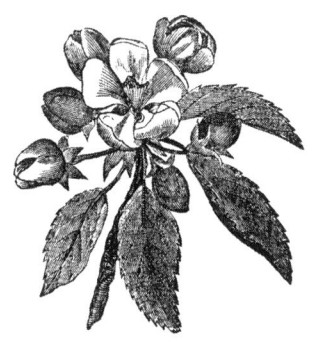

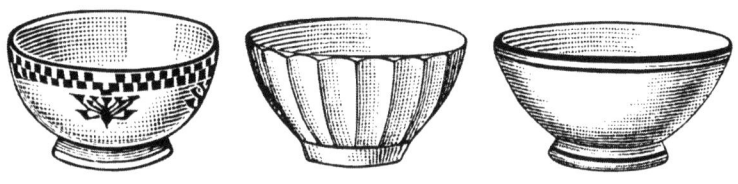

Getting Started

HANDLING NUTS AND SEEDS

Nuts and seeds should be well-sealed and stored in a cool, dry location without sunlight.

I keep nuts that are high in fats refrigerated.

I often store seeds like hemp, flax and chia in the freezer for long-term storage.

Equipment

BLENDER

When making fresh nut and seed milks, the most important kitchen appliance is a high-quality blender, with ideally 2 to 3 horse power. I have used both the VitaMix and Blendtec blenders. I recommend both of these blenders and my kitchen would not be the same without them.

Other blenders can work, however, you may need a longer blend time.

NUT MILK BAG
A quality nut milk bag, with appropriate micron mesh size, is a necessity. You can also use cheese cloth.

PERSONAL BLENDER
A personal blender comes in handy for mixing single portions and for other smaller tasks. If you don't have one, check out the Tribest Personal Blender or the Bullet.

MILK FROTHER
A good quality milk frother is great to have on hand. Frothing fresh nut milk for coffee or chai lattes adds a nice touch!

KITCHEN MISCELLANEOUS
Measuring utensils, spatulas, glass bowls, mason jars and whisks.

Soaking, Blending & Straining

SOAKING
I have spent many hours reading countless blogs and websites about the issue of soaking nuts and seeds, and I have found that there is often contradictory information regarding the duration of soak times.

I have been preparing nut milks for over ten years now. With that experience, together with the expertise of professionals I've come to respect, I will make recommendations for soak times in each chapter, as they will differ according to the nut or not be required at all.

SOAKING NUTS AND SEEDS
A soak stimulates the germination process and any enzyme inhibitors will be released into the soak water, which should then be discarded.

What are enzyme inhibitors? These special enzymes keep a seed or nut in a dormant state until conditions are right for sprouting.

By neutralizing the enzyme inhibitors, the germination growth stage is stimulated, activating the beneficial enzymes. These beneficial enzymes assist in the digestibility of nutrients.

GENERAL SOAKING PROCEDURE
Place nuts in a glass, ceramic or stainless steel bowl and rinse thoroughly. Rinse until the water runs clear.

After rinsing, cover the nuts with water.

If the weather is very hot, for longer soaks, put the nuts in the refrigerator. Otherwise, you can leave them on your counter.

After soaking, rinse until the water runs clear.

You are now ready to make milk.

Follow this process for most nuts and seeds. Each chapter will address soak times for a specific nut or seed.

BLENDING
Blending nuts with water creates a "slurry," and blending time will depend on the type of nut (or seed) and blender you are using. Keep in mind that you want to create a slurry without any detectable pieces.

Generally, I blend almonds and harder nuts for about 50 to 60 seconds in a high-powered blender and a little less for softer nuts or seeds. If you are using a blender with less than 2 horsepower, you may need to blend an additonal 30 seconds.

STRAINING THE SLURRY
After creating the slurry, place the nut milk bag in a glass Pyrex measuring cup and pour the slurry into the bag. I like

using the Pyrex measuring cup because the pouring spout makes transferring milk into serving glasses or a storage jar very easy.

When preparing 2 cups or less, I use the 4 cup Pyrex measuring cup and when I am preparing between 2 and 4 cups, I use the 8 cup Pyrex measuring cup.

You can also place the nut milk bag into a bowl or line a bowl with cheese cloth.

Squeeze all liquid from bag or cloth.

STRAINING
Straining the slurry is essential to a smooth, silky texture.

When using a high-power blender like the VitaMix or Blendtec with soft nuts like cashews and macadamias, it's optional to strain the milk. However, I recommend straining even cashew and macadamia nut milks.

To Blanche or Not to Blanche

Blanching almonds simply means to remove the brown outer skin. The traditional way of blanching is to soak almonds in boiling water for a few minutes and, when cooled, the skins come off easily.

I have found that removing the outer skin before blending does produce a milder flavor, as almond skins in high concentrations can be bitter. However, it is not necessary to blanche almonds for making milk.

If you want to blanche almonds, after soaking and rinsing place them back into the bowl and add hot water. Let them soak in the hot water for about 1 minute and the skins should easily slip off. I do not recommend boiling them.

Leftover Pulp

Many people ask me what to do with the leftover pulp after pressing the milk. Can it be used in other recipes?

Regarding almonds, I personally do not like to use leftover pulp unless the almonds were blanched. Pulp from unblanched almonds has a tendency to be bitter and, in large concentrations, can be hard on digestion.

The softer nuts without brown skins, like cashews and macadamias, leave a lovely paste after the milk press. These pastes are more ideal for use in preparing additional recipes.

Milk Storage & Shelf Life

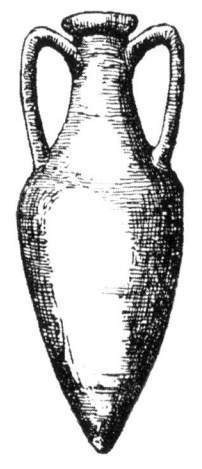

My favorite way to store freshly made milk is using a glass jar with a tight-fitting lid. Refrigerate immediately and it should last 3 to 5 days.

Without an emulsifying agent, the milk will naturally separate.

No worries, just give it a good shake!

Lastly, experiment—let your intuition and taste buds guide you!

> **Caution:**
> Some people have allergies to certain nuts and seeds. Consult with your physician if you have any concerns. Plant-based milks may not be appropriate for infants.

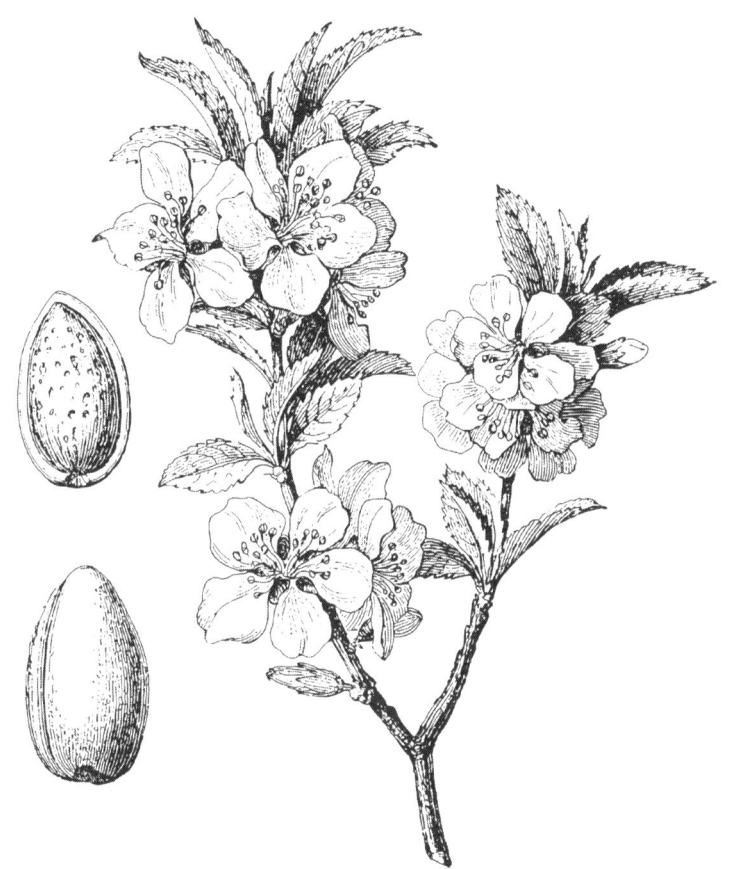

Almonds

Wild almonds are said to have originated in western Asia, eventually spreading into the Mediterranean region before Franciscan Padres brought the almond tree to California by way of Spain around the late 1600s.

The coastal weather did not provide the optimal growing environment for the almond trees, and it wasn't until one hundred years later that research and crossbreeding helped develop several of today's almond varieties.

By the turn of the 20th century the almond industry was firmly established in the Sacramento and San Joaquin areas of California's great Central Valley, and the United States has since become the dominant supplier of almonds.

Almonds are a high source of vitamin E, calcium, magnesium and potassium. Additionally, they are a source of protein, are high in fiber and low in sugars.

Almond Soak Time:
approximately 8 to 10 hours
Discard soak water

If you decide to soak your almonds longer than 10 hours, I recommend you rinse the water after 10 to 12 hours.

Simple Unsweetened Almond Milk

Your basic, unsweetened milk.
Use raw, unflavored almonds.

If the slurry produced by the blending of water and nuts is not properly strained, you will get bits of pulp, peel or a fine sediment in the finished product. To create a smooth texture without sediment, it's important to strain the slurry using a nut milk bag or cheese cloth.

- *Soaking will increase bulk.*
- *All recipes call for a dry measurement of the nut, before soaking.*
- *Using more almonds produces a richer milk and also provides a stronger almond flavor.*
- *Recipes can be cut in half or doubled.*

There are a wide range of proportions that you can use when making almond milk, and I encourage you to try a few different ratios.

These recipes range from creating a thick, full-bodied milk by using a larger ratio of almonds to water, to a light blend with a small ratio of nuts to water.

The blends that use fewer almonds can be fortified with excellent nutritional supplements that bring both body and taste to the milks.

RECOMMENDED USES

Full bodied blends: for milk, custards, ice creams, vegan cheeses, savory sauces, foaming or pouring for coffee, tea and soda fountain creams.

Medium blends: for milk, custard, cereal, granola, oatmeal, smoothie bases, foaming or pouring for coffee, tea and soda fountain creams.

Light blends: for cereal, granola, oatmeal and milkshake bases.

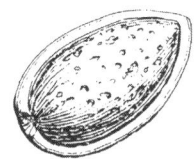

Almond Milk Ratios

Almond Milk — Thicker, Full Body
One quart

- 4 cups filtered water
- 2 cups almonds

Blend well.
Strain.

Almond Milk — Creamy, Full Body
One quart

    4   cups filtered water
    1 ¾ cups almonds

Blend well.
Strain.

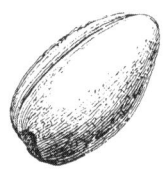

Almond Milk — Full Body
One quart

    4   cups filtered water
    1 ½ cups almonds

Blend well.
Strain.

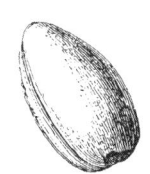

Almond Milk — Full to Medium Body
One quart

    4   cups filtered water
    1 ¼ cups almonds

Blend well.
Strain.

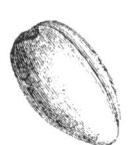

Almond Milk — Medium Body
One quart

    4   cups filtered water
    1   cup almonds

Blend well.
Strain.

Almond Milk — Medium Body to Light Body
One quart

    4   cups filtered water
    ¾   cup almonds

Blend well.
Strain.

Almond Milk — Light Body
One quart

Using lecithin and tocotrienols will provide body and reduce separation.

The tocotrienols also add a hint of sweetness.

    4   cups filtered water
    ½   cup almonds
    3   Tablespoons tocotrienols
    2   Tablespoons non-GMO lecithin

Blend almonds and water.
Strain.
Pour milk back into a clean blender.
Add lecithin and tocotrienols.
Blend well.

Almond Milk — Light Body
One Quart

This recipe uses only ¼ cup of almonds to a quart of filtered water and produces a very light milk! This blend works well for pouring over cereal or granola, and I use this as a base for milkshakes. To provide more flavor for such a light milk, try adding sweetener of choice and vanilla.

Using lecithin, tocotrienols and chicory will provide body, reduce separation and add a hint of sweetness.

  4   cups filtered water
  ¼   cup almonds
  3   Tablespoons tocos
  3   Tablespoons chicory powder
  2   Tablespoons non-GMO organic lecithin
  1   Tablespoon honey or coconut palm sugar (optional)
  1   teaspoon vanilla extract (optional)

Blend almonds and water.
Strain.
Pour milk back into a clean blender.
Add lecithin, tocotrienols, chicory, and optional sweetener and vanilla.
Blend well.

Milk from Almond Butter
One quart

Many people have asked me about using almond butter for making milk. I rarely use almond butter to make milk, because somehow the flavor is never right for me—but in a pinch it can work.

  4   cups filtered water
  ½   cup almond butter

Blend well.
Strain.

HOW LONG DOES IT LAST?

Keep your milk in a tightly sealed glass jar in a cold refrigerator. The milk should last 3 to 5 days.

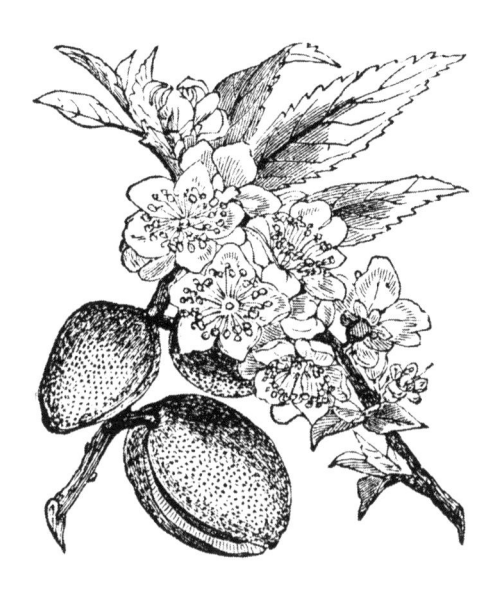

Fruit Sweetened Almond Milks

- All of the almond measurements are dry, pre-soaked measurements.
- The sweetened recipes contained in this section are primarily sweetened with dried fruits and fruit juices. Use organic whenever possible.
- The blends with bananas (fresh or frozen) and fresh vegetables are best consumed immediately or within a day.
- Quart recipes can be cut in half or reduced for a smaller portion, and the individual servings can be doubled for a larger portion.

TIP: *Keep some pre-soaked almonds in the freezer for quick individual servings.*

Make sure they are not wet when you put them into the freezer.

WHEN USING DRIED FRUIT

OPTION 1

Most recipes are based on this procedure.

- Add all ingredients to the blender. Blend on high so the nuts and dried fruits are broken down. Then strain.

- **EXCEPTION!** Always blend banana and fresh fruits into the milk after it has been strained.

OPTION 2

This option is if you prefer to have blended pieces of dried fruit in your milk blend.

- Prepare the almond milk, then pour the milk back into a clean blender. Add the dried fruit and blend well. This will add more texture by leaving bits of dried fruit in the milk.

- I use this method when I want a smoothie consistency.

Date Almond Milk

One quart

    4   cups filtered water
    1 ¼ cups almonds
    2   medjool dates, medium/large, pitted

Add all ingredients to blender.
Blend well; dates should be well broken down.
Strain.
If you prefer a sweeter milk, add more dates.
Dates are mild in flavor and enhance the sweetness of the milk rather than adding a complex layer of flavor.

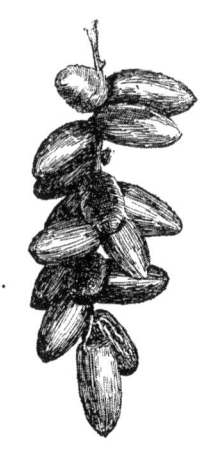

Generally, medjool dates are moist and it's unnecessary to soak the dates first. If you are using dates that have less moisture, consider soaking for a few hours so that they will easily blend into the slurry.

Honey Almond Milk
One quart

For those of you who love the taste of raw honey—and who doesn't—this is a simple, tasty recipe.

- 4 cups filtered water
- 1 ¼ cups almonds
- 1 ½ Tablespoons raw honey or to taste

Add all ingredients to blender.
Blend well.
Strain.

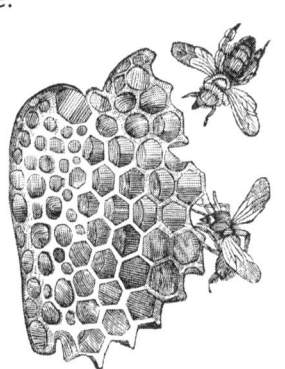

Apple Almond Milk
One quart

Simple and delicious.

Using one cup of water cuts the sweetness and provides a more subtle flavor. However, if you prefer a sweeter apple flavor, use a full quart of apple juice and omit the water.

- 3 cups organic apple juice
- 1 cup filtered water
- 1 ½ cups almonds

Add all ingredients to blender.
Blend well.
Strain.

Note: Seasonal organic pear juice can be substituted.

Apple Lime Almond Milk
One quart

This is surprisingly delicious. Try pouring over crushed ice and add a sprig of mint

- 4 cups organic apple juice
- 1 ½ cups almonds
- 1 ¼ Tablespoons lime zest
- 1 ¼ Tablespoons lime juice

Add all ingredients to blender.
Blend well.
Strain.

TIP: *For such a small amount of zest, use a potato peeler to take off the lime rind and press that into the measuring spoon.*

Pear & Candied Ginger Almond Milk
16 ounces

- 2 cups pear juice
- ¾ cup almonds
- 1 ½ Tablespoons candied ginger or to taste*

Rough chop the candied ginger into small pieces.
Add all ingredients to blender.
Blend well.
Strain.

*You can also substitute fresh ginger by using 1 tablespoon roughly chopped, or to taste.

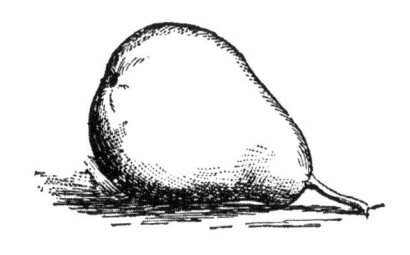

Cranberry Almond Milk
One quart

    4   cups filtered water
    1 ¼ cups almonds
    1   cup dried cranberries

Add all ingredients to blender.
Blend well.
Strain.

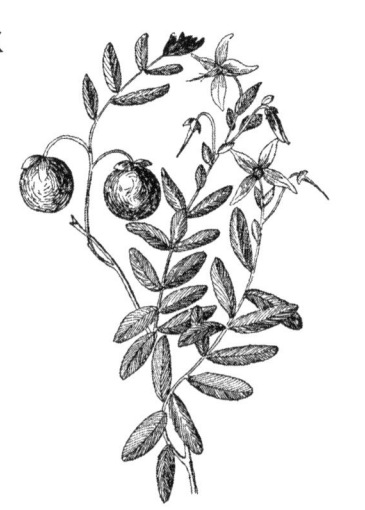

Sweet & Sour Gooseberry Almond Milk
(also known as Golden Berry)
One quart

    4   cups filtered water
    1 ¼ cups almonds
    1   cup dried gooseberries
    1   Tablespoon raw honey

Add all ingredients to blender.
Blend well.
Strain.

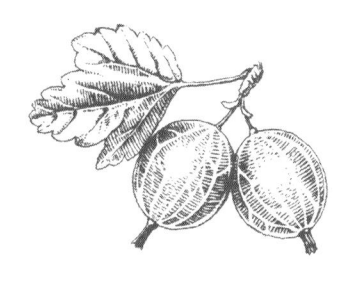

Maple Orange Almond Milk
One quart

- 4 cups filtered water
- 1 ¼ cups almonds
- ¼ cup maple syrup
- 1 teaspoon organic orange extract

Add all ingredients to blender.
Blend well.
Strain.

Raisin Cinnamon Almond Milk
One quart

- 4 cups filtered water
- 1 ¼ cups almonds
- 1 cup raisins
- ½ teaspoon cinnamon

Add all ingredients to blender.
Blend well.
Strain.

Banana Fig Almond Smoothie
Single 8 ounce serving

- 1 cup filtered water
- ¼ cup almonds
- ⅓ cup dried figs*
- ½ cup banana, fresh or frozen

Blend almonds and water.
Strain.
Pour milk back into a clean blender.
Add figs and banana.
Blend well.

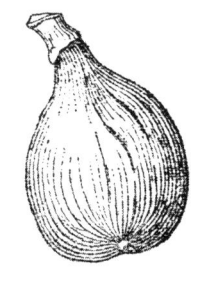

* If the figs are moist, it's unnecessary to soak them first. For figs with less moisture, consider soaking for a few hours so they will easily blend into the smoothie.

Pineapple Ginger Almond Milk
Single 10 ounce serving

- 1 cup pineapple juice
- ¼ cup filtered water
- ⅓ cup almonds
- ½ Tablespoon fresh chopped ginger, or to taste

Add all ingredients to blender.
Blend well.
Strain.

Pineapple Orange Apricot Almond Milk
Single 10 ounce serving

- 1 cup pineapple juice
- ¼ cup filtered water
- ⅓ cup almonds
- 2 Tablespoons fresh orange juice
- 3 dried apricots *
- ½ teaspoon orange zest

Add all ingredients to blender.
Blend well
Strain.

* If the apricots are moist, it's unnecessary to soak them first. For apricots with less moisture, consider soaking for a few hours so they will easily blend into the slurry.

TIP: *For such a small amount of zest, use a potato peeler to take off the orange rind and press that into the measuring spoon.*

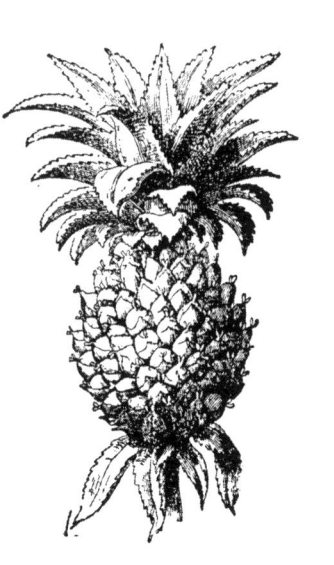

> **OPTIONAL**
>
> If you prefer to have apricot pieces in your milk as opposed to a smooth texture:
>
> > Blend juice, water, almonds and zest.
> > Strain.
> > Pour milk back into a clean blender.
> > Add apricots.
> > Blend well.

Goji Berry Pomegranate Honey Almond Milk

Single 8 ounce serving

- 1 cup filtered water
- ½ cup pomegranate seeds, fresh or frozen
- ¼ cup almonds
- 2 Tablespoons goji berries
- 1 teaspoon raw honey

Blend all ingredients well.
Strain.

Prune Almond Milk

Single 10 ounce serving

- 1 ¼ cups filtered water
- ¼ cup almonds
- ¼ cup chopped prunes
- 1 teaspoon honey (optional)

Place all ingredients in blender.
Blend well.
Strain.

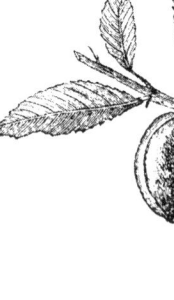

MILKS ALIVE

Prune & Candied Ginger Almond Milk
Single 10 ounce serving

- 1 ¼ cups filtered water
- ¼ cup almonds
- ¼ cup chopped prunes
- 1 Tablespoon candied ginger, or to taste

Place all ingredients in blender.
Blend well.
Strain.

Prune Banana & Ginger Almond Smoothie
Single 12 ounce serving

- 1 ½ cups filtered water
- ¼ cup almonds
- ¼ cup chopped prunes
- ½ cup banana, fresh or frozen
- 1 Tablespoon candied ginger, or to taste

Blend almonds and water. Strain.
Pour milk back into a clean blender.
Add prunes, ginger and banana.
Blend well.

Carrot Almond Milk
16 ounces

Prepare fresh carrot juice or substitute store bought.

- 1 ½ cups carrot juice
- ½ cup filtered water
- ½ cup almonds

Add all ingredients to blender.
Blend well. Strain.

Carrot Pineapple Almond Milk
16 ounces

Prepare the almond carrot milk.

    1   cup almond carrot milk
    1   cup pineapple juice

Blend.

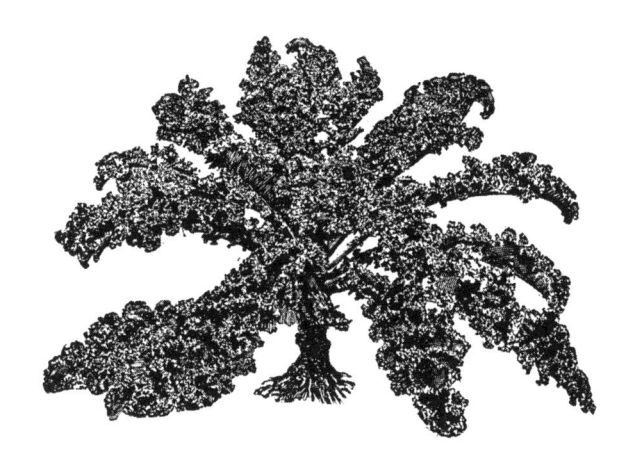

Kale Recipes

Remove the stems and coursely chop the kale. For measurement gently press the kale down into the measuring cup.

Kale Apple Almond Milk
16 ounces

    1 ½ cups apple juice
    ½   cup filtered water
    ⅓   cup almonds
    1   cup kale, stemmed and coursely chopped

Add all ingredients to blender.
Blend well.
Strain.

Kale Apple & Fresh Ginger Almond Milk
16 ounces

- 1 ½ cups apple juice
- ½ cup filtered water
- 1 cup kale, stemmed and coursely chopped
- ⅓ cup almonds
- 1 Tablespoon fresh ginger, or to taste

Add all ingredients to blender.
Blend well.
Strain.

Kale Celery Apple Almond Milk
16 ounces

- 1 ½ cups apple juice
- ½ cup filtered water
- ½ cup almonds
- 1 cup kale, stemmed and coursely chopped
- ½ cup celery
- 1 Tablespoon fresh ginger, or to taste (optional)

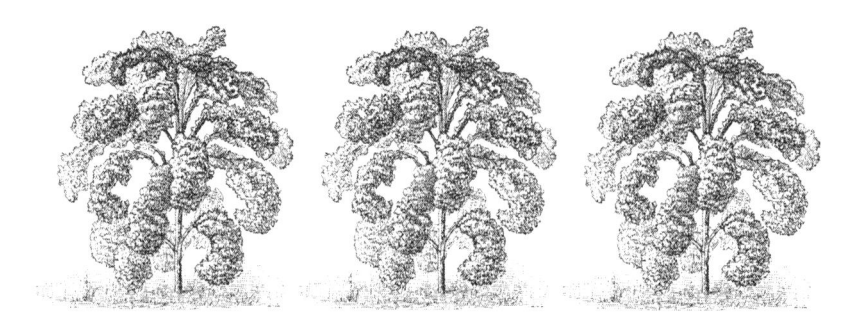

Add all ingredients to blender.
Blend well.
Strain.

Kale Pear Banana & Seed Mix Almond Smoothie

16 ounces

- 1 ½ cups pear juice*
- ½ cup filtered water
- ⅓ cup almonds
- 1 cup kale, stemmed and coursely chopped
- ½ cup banana, fresh or frozen
- 1 Tablespoon fresh ginger, or to taste
- 1 teaspoon chia seeds
- 1 teaspoon flax seeds

Blend almonds, water, pear juice, kale and ginger.
Strain.
Pour milk back into a clean blender.
Add flax, chai seed and banana.
Blend well.

* You can substitute apple juice

Kale Apple Banana Hemp & Almond Smoothie

16 ounces

- 1 ½ cups apple juice
- ½ cup filtered water
- ⅓ cup almonds
- ¾ cup kale, stemmed and coursely chopped
- ½ cup banana, fresh or frozen
- 2 Tablespoons hemp seeds
- 2 teaspoons tocotrienols
- 2 teaspoons chicory
- 1 teaspoon lecithin

Blend almonds, juice, water, and kale.
Strain.
Pour milk back into a clean blender.
Add banana, hemp, tocos, chicory and lecithin.
Blend well.

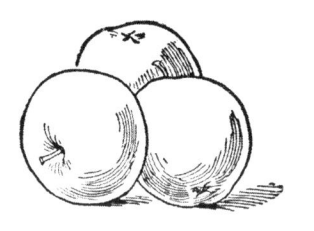

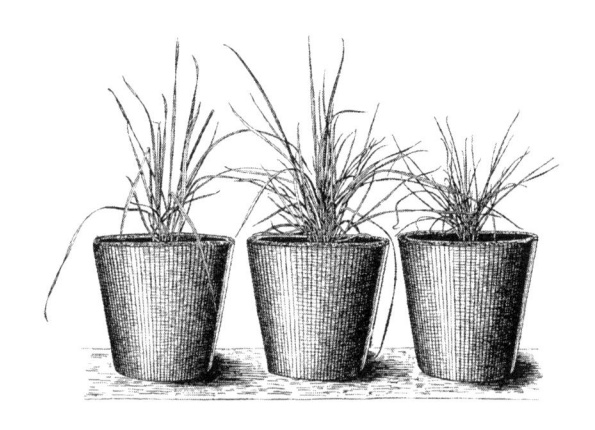

Wheatgrass recipes

- You can find 4" by 4" potted containers of wheatgrass in your health food store.

- By sight, cut ⅓ to ½ of the wheatgrass growing in a 4" by 4" container.

- If you are growing wheatgrass in a large flat, measure out a 4" by 4" section, and cut approximately ⅓ to ½ of the 4" by 4" square.

Wheatgrass Kale Apple Almond Milk
16 ounces

2	cups apple juice
¼	cup almonds
¼	cup kale, stemmed and coursely chopped
⅓	4" by 4" container of wheatgrass
1	teaspoon tocotrienols
1	teaspoon lecithin
1	teaspoon chicory

Blend apple juice, almonds, kale and wheatgrass.
Strain.
Pour milk back into a clean blender.
Add tocos, lecithin and chicory.
Blend well.

Wheatgrass Kale Apple Lime Almond Milk

16 ounces

- 2 cups apple juice
- ¼ cup almonds
- ⅓ cup kale, stemmed and coursely chopped
- ⅓ 4" by 4" container of wheatgrass
- 2 teaspoons lime juice
- ½ teaspoon lime zest

Blend well.
Strain.

TIP: *For such a small amount of zest, use a potato peeler to take off the lime rind and press that into the measuring spoon.*

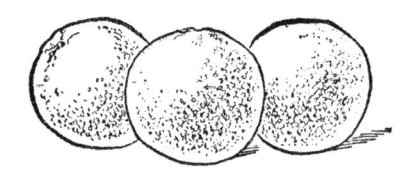

Wheatgrass Kale Orange Almond Milk

16 ounces

- 2 cups filtered water
- ⅓ cup unsweetened, organic orange juice concentrate
- ¼ cup almonds
- ¼ cup kale, stemmed and coursely chopped
- ⅓ 4" by 4" container of wheatgrass
- ¼ teaspoon stevia

Add all ingredients to blender.
Blend well.
Strain.

Wheatgrass Kale Celery Apple Almond Milk

18 ounces

- 1 ¾ cups apple juice
- ½ cup filtered water
- 1 cup kale, stemmed and coursely chopped
- ⅓ 4" by 4" container wheatgrass
- ½ cup celery
- ⅓ cup almonds
- 1 ½ teaspoons tocotrienols
- 1 ½ teaspoons lecithin

Blend juice, almonds, water, kale, wheatgrass and celery.
Strain.
Pour milk back into a clean blender.
Add tocos and lecithin.
Blend well.

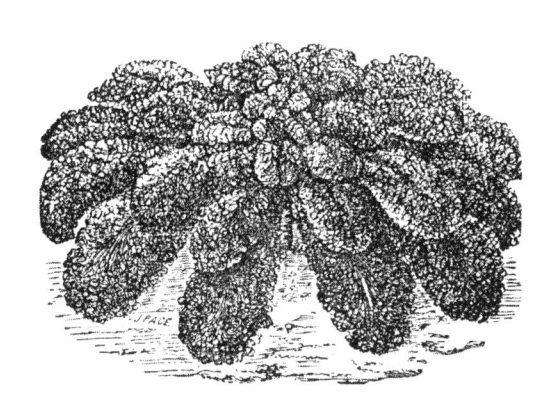

Wheatgrass Kale Celery Lemon Apple & Ginger Almond Milk

18 ounces

- 1 ¾ cups apple juice
- ½ cup filtered water
- 1 cup kale, stemmed and coursely chopped
- ⅓ 4" by 4" container wheatgrass
- ½ cup celery
- ⅓ cup almonds
- 2 Tablespoons lemon juice
- 1 Tablespoon candied ginger or to taste - optional
- 1 ½ teaspoons tocotrienols
- 1 ½ teaspoons lecithin

Blend juice, water, kale, wheatgrass, celery and almonds.
Strain.
Pour milk back into a clean blender.
Add lemon juice, ginger, tocos and lecithin.
Blend well.

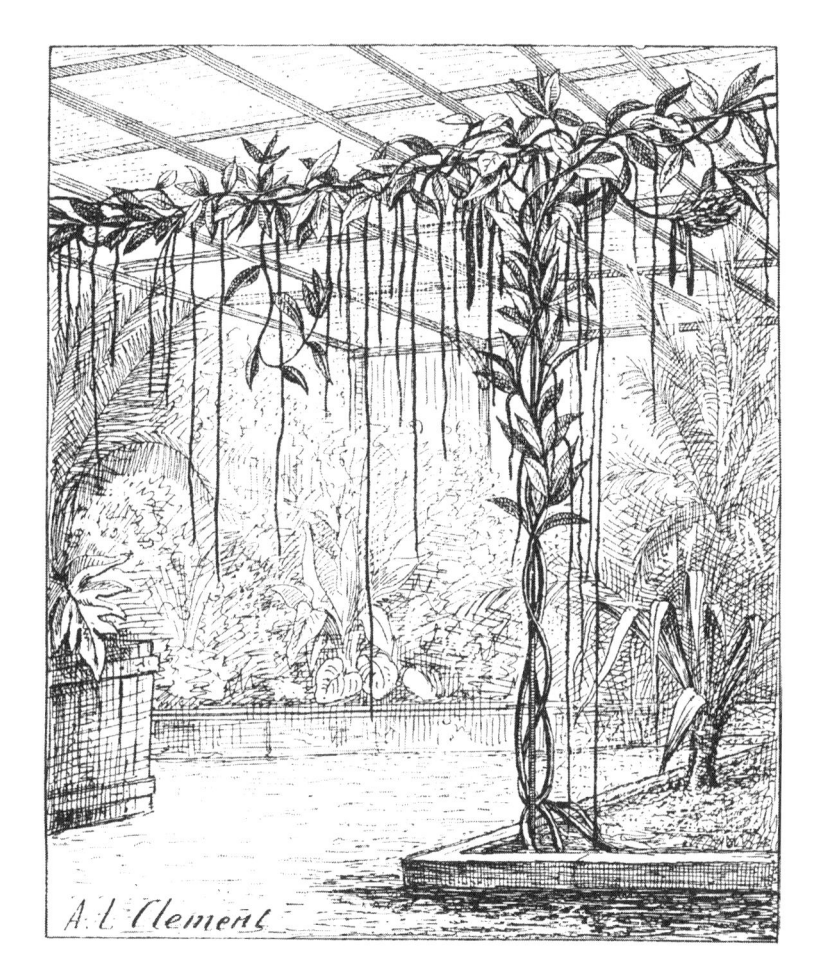

Vanilla

The intoxicating fragrance of vanilla...

When Milks Alive was selling at local farmers markets, our vanilla blends were extrememly popular. Customers who told me they never liked carob become carob lovers and the Orange Blossom was one of our big hits!

Besides the love we put into preparing our milks, our recipe using homemade "vanilla liquid," coconut butter and a pinch of Himalayan salt made our vanilla milk blends very special.

Fresh Vanilla Liquid

Making your own vanilla liquid is easy, aromatic and flavorful, without using any alcohol and can be used in any recipe that calls for vanilla.

Keep this refrigerated in a glass bottle and it will be good for about 6 weeks.

There will be separation; it's necessary to shake well before each use.

    5   vanilla beans
    2 ¼ cups filtered water

Vanilla beans should be pliable to the touch (good moisture content) as opposed to dry and brittle. If they are hard, they are too old or have not been stored properly to use for making fresh vanilla.

PREPARATION:

- Cut off the tips of the vanilla beans.
- Cut the vanilla beans into small pieces, using the whole bean.
- Add the vanilla beans and about half the filtered water into the blender.
- Use a low speed and slowly increase to high.
- Stop the blender and pour about half the remaining water down the sides of the blender to get all those precious seeds down into the mixture.
- Blend again, using a low speed and slowly increase to high.
- Add the rest of the filtered water down the sides of the blender.
- Use a spatula, on the inside of the blender, to scrape all the vanilla beans into your vanilla mixture.

WHEN MAKING VANILLA MILK:

For a full flavor, I recommend using the dry measurement of 1 ¼ cups of almonds, before soaking, to make 1 quart of vanilla almond milk.

Also, prepare the fresh vanilla liquid ahead of time.

NOT USING FRESH VANILLA LIQUID?
Use the following:

- Vanilla extract, ¾ teaspoon to 1 quart of almond milk.
- Pure ground vanilla beans, ⅛ teaspoon to 1 quart of almond milk.

Vanilla Almond Milk
One quart

First, prepare a quart of plain almond milk and fresh vanilla liquid (or use vanilla extract or pure ground vanilla beans, as specified above).

- 4 cups almond milk
- 2 Tablespoons light, unflavored agave
- 1 ½ Tablespoons liquid vanilla (or one of the other specified options)
- 1 ½ Tablespoons coconut butter
- 1 Tablespoon powdered non GMO lecithin (optional)*
- Pinch of Pink Himalayan salt

Add all ingredients to blender.

Blend well to break down the coconut butter and disperse the lecithin.

Strain. There will be sediment from the coconut butter, so strain for the creamiest texture.

*Lecithin acts as an emulsifier, preventing separation, and will also add body to the milk. Make sure you are using a non-GMO powdered lecithin.

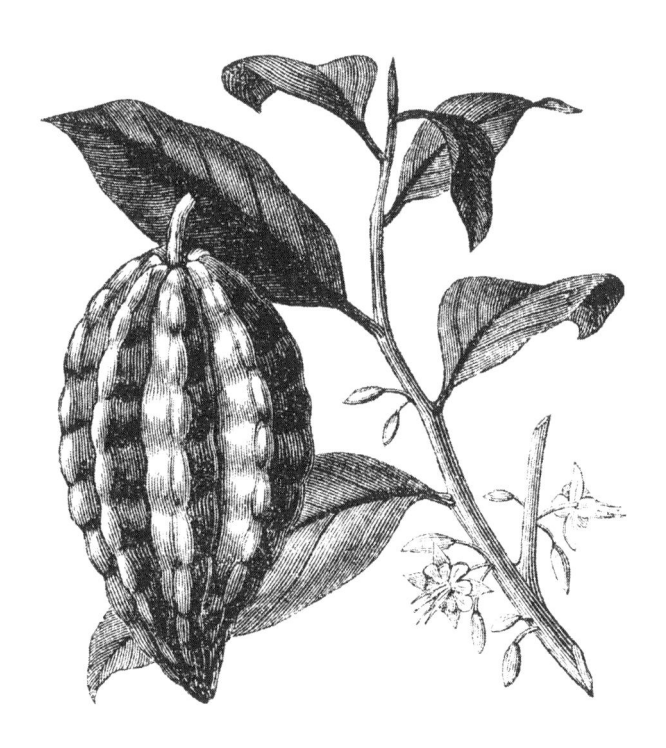

Chocolate Almond Milk
One quart

Prepare one quart of vanilla almond milk.

- 4 cups vanilla almond milk.
- 2 tablespoon powdered cacao or unsweetened chocolate
- 2 teaspoons agave

Blend well.

Hot Chocolate
Place individual chocolate almond milk serving into your frother or gently heat on the stove.

Chocolate Peppermint Almond Milk
16 ounces

Prepare the chocolate almond milk.

    2   cups chocolate almond milk
    ¼   teaspoon peppermint oil

Blend.

Mesquite Chocolate Malt Almond Milk
16 ounces

Prepare the vanilla almond milk.

    2   cups vanilla almond milk
    1   Tablespoon powered cacao or unsweetened chocolate
    2 ¼ teaspoons mesquite powder
    1   teaspoon agave

Blend well.

Carob Almond Milk
One quart

Prepare one quart of vanilla almond milk.

    4   cups vanilla almond milk
    2   Tablespoons carob powder (raw or roasted)
    2   teaspoons agave

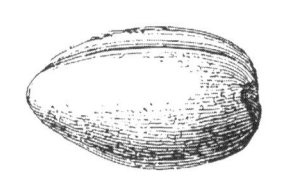

Blend well.

Carob Malted Almond Milk

Single 8 ounce serving

If you love malt flavor, you must try this one!

Prepare the vanilla almond milk.

- 1 cup vanilla almond milk
- 2 teaspoons carob powder (raw or roasted)
- 1 teaspoon maca powder
- 1 teaspoon mesquite powder
- ½ teaspoon agave

Blend well.

Carob Malted Almond Smoothie

Single 8 ounce serving

Prepare the carob malted almond milk.

- 1 cup carob malted almond milk
- ½ cup banana fresh or frozen

Blend well.

IDEAS:

You can substitute chocolate for the carob in the Carob Malted Milk and Carob Malted Smoothie recipes!

You can substitute carob for the chocolate in the Chocolate Peppermint Milk recipe!

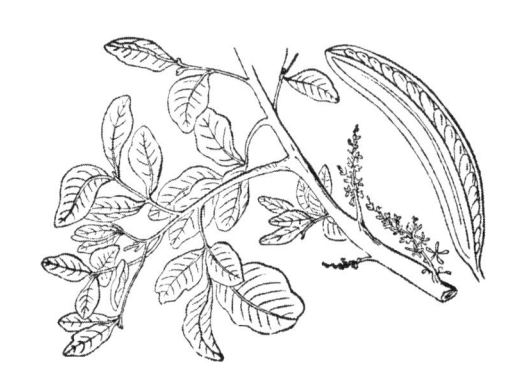

Orange Blossom Almond Milk
One quart

- 4 cups vanilla almond milk
- 1 ½ Tablespoons freshly grated organic orange zest
- 1 ½ teaspoons agave

Blend well to incorporate the orange zest flavor. Strain to remove the orange zest from the milk.

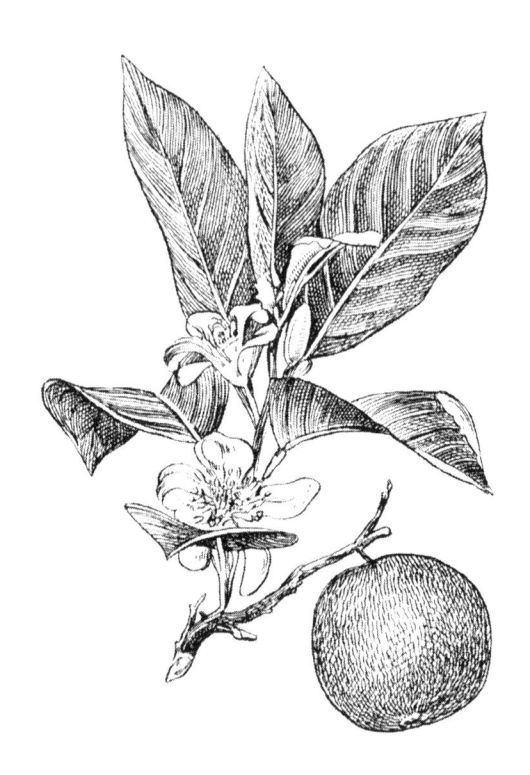

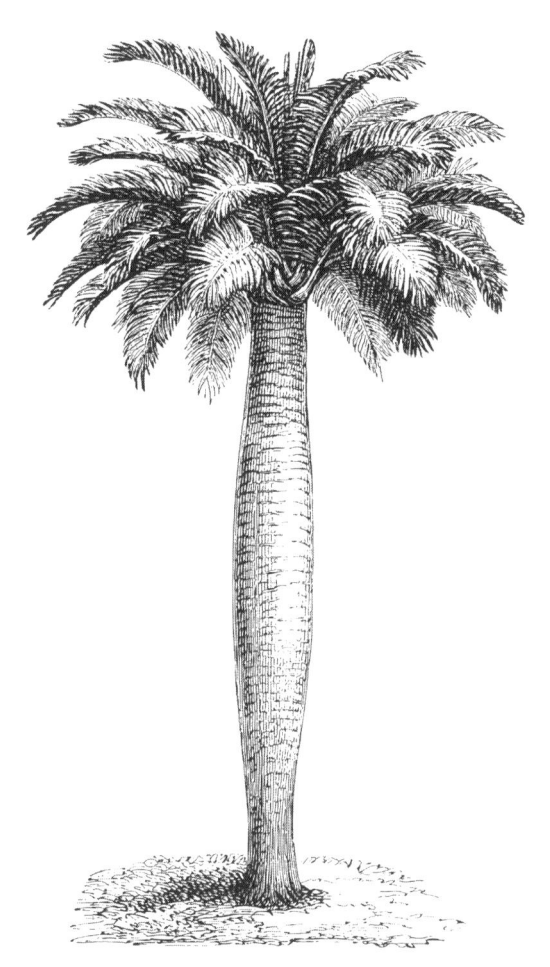

Coconuts

Coconuts are delicious and nutritious!

A common misconception is that coconuts are high in fats, clog arteries and raise cholesterol levels.

It's important to recognize that some saturated fats are healthy and essential for us, while others are not. There are small, medium and long chain saturated fats and it is the *long chain fatty acids* that store fats and are associated with the "bad" cholesterol. It is the *medium chain fatty acids*, that are found in coconuts, which are easy to digest and are a source of fuel and energy.

Coconuts are also rich in lauric acid, which is known for being antiviral, antibacterial and antifungal. Lauric acid is naturally occurring in human breast milk, assisting infants in fighting off bacteria and viruses. Coconuts are also high in fiber, magnesium, copper, iron and selenium.

Virgin coconut oil is used for making natural soaps and other health products and is one of the healthiest products that we can put on our skin.

So, set your sails! Lush tropical flavors, aromas and tastes await...

Young Thai Coconut Milk

The recipes in this chapter all use young Thai coconuts. The flesh of the young Thai coconut is easy to work with and it makes great milk.

Our discerning, coconut-loving customers would line up early at the market, knowing that our coconut blends would sell out within a few hours of opening. They truly appreciated that we made fresh coconut milk and I've had many people tell me they were addicted to our coconut milks!

Making fresh coconut milk does take extra time and it is well worth the effort. I recommend that you buy several coconuts and make enough milk to keep some frozen. Fresh coconut milk will freeze very well, unlike canned coconut milk. It should last for several weeks in the freezer, but chances are it will never last that long!

- Open the coconut.
- Drain the coconut water.
- Scoop out the coconut flesh.
- Blend the coconut water and flesh.

STEP 1 - OPEN THE COCONUT

Always inspect the coconut once it is opened. The coconut meat should be white without any discolorations and the water should have a clear to opalescent look.

When opening Young Thai coconuts, it is best to use a strong, forged meat cleaver. With an intentional motion, swing the cleaver down on the top of the coconut. Do this several times to create a circle or a square. Each swing of the cleaver should penetrate the shell of the coconut. Then use the tip of the cleaver to pry the top off.

STEP 2 - DRAIN THE COCONUT WATER:

Drain the coconut water into a bowl.

Once you've opened the coconuts that you're using, strain the water through cheese cloth or a nut milk bag to remove any coconut shards.

Refrigerate your coconut water while you are scooping out the flesh of the coconut.

STEP 3 - SCOOP OUT THE COCONUT FLESH

Lay the coconut on its side and with a strong swing of the cleaver, halve the coconut. This makes scooping out the flesh very easy, especially if the opening that you've created at the top is small.

Use a strong spoon to remove the inner white flesh. The flesh of the coconut will vary in both texture and feel. It can vary from translucent and soft to compact and dense. It's best to scoop out large sections instead of small tiny pieces, as larger pieces are easier to clean.

Place the flesh in a colander. With a paring knife, remove any leftover shards.

Once all the meat is cleaned, you are ready to make the fresh coconut milk.

Fresh Coconut Milk

One quart

This delectable, nutrient-packed milk from fresh coconuts can be used from soups to desserts.

 4 cups fresh young Thai coconut water
 20 ounces coconut flesh, approximately 2 ¼ cups

This will produce a thick coconut milk. Do not dilute it; it will be a perfect when added to the almond milk and it makes very creamy desserts.

Blend until creamy. If the coconut meat was thicker, blend for a longer time. Blend until you get a creamy milk with all the coconut meat dissolved. It should have a smooth texture.

TIP: *If you are making enough milk to store some in the freezer, I suggest that you store in smaller portions and only defrost what you need.*

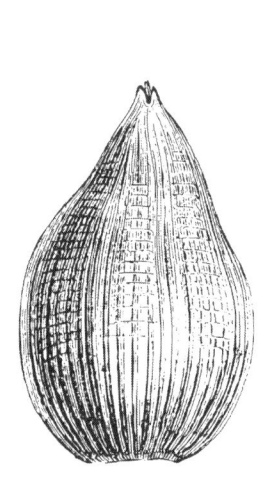

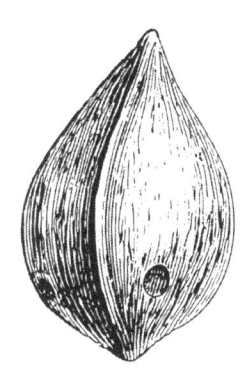

FOR THE ALMOND COCONUT MILK:

1) Prepare your almond milk. I recommend the dry measurement of 1 ¼ cups of almonds to a quart of water.
2) Prepare your coconut milk or you may substitue canned coconut milk.

Almond Coconut Milk
One quart

    2 ½ cups unsweetened almond milk
    1 ½ cups fresh young Thai coconut milk

Add almond milk and coconut milk to blender.
Blend well.

Coco Loco
One quart

    4   cups fresh coconut water
    1 ½ cups almonds

Do not add sweetener! You will be surprised how sweet and delicious this is.
Blend well.
Strain.

Coco Loco Supreme
One quart

This blend does not use any filtered water, only almonds, coconut water and coconut meat.

First prepare both the Coco Loco blend and the fresh coconut milk.

    2 ½ cups Coco Loco blend
    1 ½ cups fresh coconut milk

Blend well.

Pina Colada
One quart

    2   cups almond coconut milk
    2   cups pineapple juice
    1 ½ Tablespoon coconut sugar or agave (optional)

Add almond coconut milk and pineapple juice to blender, with optional sweetener.
Blend well.

I have done this with freshly made pineapple juice, and it's a ticket to heaven!

More often, I will buy organic, unsweetened pineapple juice and it works really well. Just add a small amount of sweetener if necessary.

Pineapple Banana Colada Smoothie
Single 8 ounce serving

    1   cup Pina Colada blend
    ½   cup banana, fresh or frozen

Blend well.

Pineapple Banana Ginger Colada Smoothie
Single 8 ounce serving

    1   cup Pina Colada blend
    ½   cup banana, fresh or frozen
    1   Tablespoon candied ginger, or to taste

Blend well.

Coconut Milk from Dry, Shredded Coconut

Here is another option for making coconut milk.

After blending allow the mixture to cool before straining.

    2 ⅔ cups dry unsweetened shredded coconut
    2 ½ cups hot water

Blend the shredded coconut and 2 cups of hot water.
This is a thick mixture.
Allow it to cool.
Pour the mixture into your filter bag.
Use the remaining ½ cup of water to pour down the sides of the blender.
Using a spatula, bring all the coconut down into the blender.
Pour the remaining mixture into the filter bag.
Strain.

Coconut meal left from the pressing can be used in crackers, crusts, cookies and homemade granola.

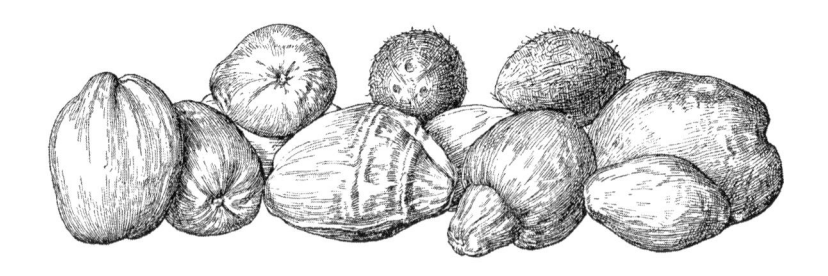

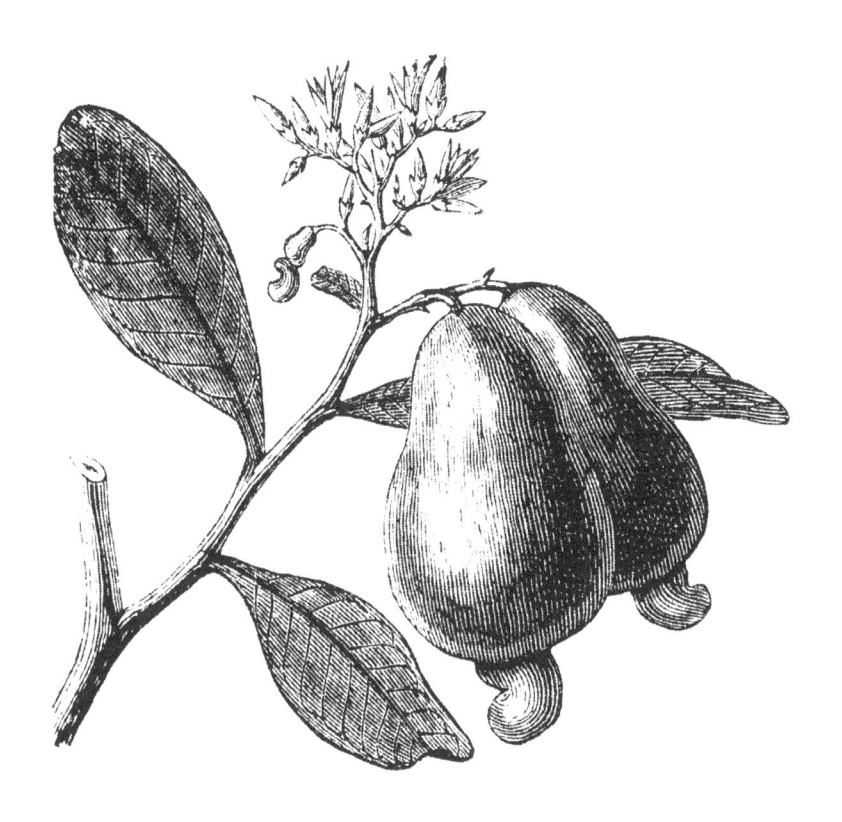

Cashews

Cashew trees, native to Brazil, are now widely grown in warm, tropical climates. The cashew nut grows at the bottom of an edible fruit known as the "cashew apple," which looks very much like a pear. The cashew apple is used as a drink and also fermented into a liquor.

Cashews are a good source of antioxidants and trace minerals such as copper, iron and zinc. Cashews are also lower in fat than many nuts and about 85% is oleic acid, which is the heart-healthy fat found in olive oil.

Approximately 10% of their weight is from starch, which is a characteristic that makes cashews very effective in bringing "body" to vegan culinary creations—including milk, desserts, cheeses and savory recipes.

Milk made from cashews has a very subtle, almost neutral flavor, which allows it to blend well with other ingredients. Proportions are important; using too many nuts can create a "chalky" taste.

Although blending cashews and water will not produce much sediment, I still recommend that you strain the milk! It is a simple and easy step as there is a lot less pulp than other nuts. Straining the blend will produce a very creamy milk.

Cashew Soak Time:
approximately 3 to 4 hours

Discard soak water

Simple Cashew Milk
16 ounces

- 2 cups filtered water
- ½ cup cashews

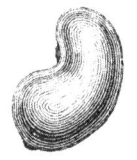

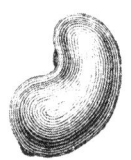

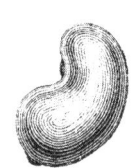

Blend well.
Strain.

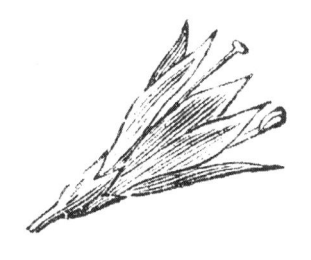

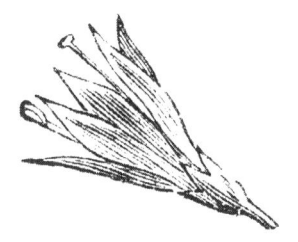

Sweet Cashew Milk

16 ounces

Coconut palm sugar compliments cashews really well.

- 2 cups filtered water
- ½ cup cashews
- 1 ½ Tablespoons coconut palm sugar

Blend well.
Strain.

Creamy Cashew Coconut Milk

Single 8 ounce serving

- 1 cup plain cashew milk
- 2 Tablespoons coconut milk
- 2 teaspoons coconut palm sugar

Blend well.

Cashew Almond Date Milk

16 ounces

- 2 cups filtered water
- ¼ cup cashews
- ¼ cup almonds
- 2 medjool dates, medium/large, pitted

Blend well.
Strain.

Vegan Egg Nog
16 ounces

Yum, rich and creamy!

- 2 cups filtered water
- ⅓ cup cashews
- ⅓ cup macadamia nuts (do not soak)
- 2 Tablespoons coconut milk
- 3 Tablespoons coconut palm sugar
- 1 Tablespoon fresh avocado
- ¼ cup banana, fresh or frozen (optional)
- ⅓ teaspoon vanilla extract
- ⅓ teaspoon cinnamon
- ⅛ teaspoon ground nutmeg
- pinch of Himalayan sea salt

Note: If you don't have a ⅓ teaspoon measurement, use a heaping ¼ teaspoon.

Blend water, macadamia nuts and cashews.
Strain.
Pour milk back into a clean blender.
Add remaining ingredients.
Blend well.

Cashew Hemp Milk
16 ounces

The cashews cut the strong flavor of hemp.

- 2 cups filtered water
- ½ cup cashews
- ⅓ cup organic, shelled hemp seeds

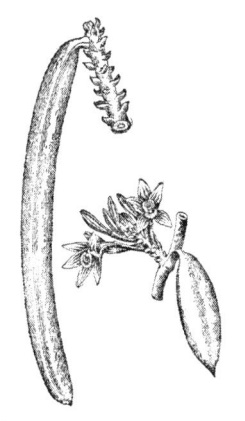

Blend well.
Strain.

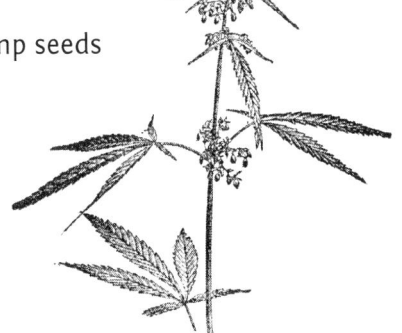

Cashew Hemp Chocolate Milk

Single 8 ounce serving

Cocoa, cacao powder or chocolate syrup can be used. If using sweetened chocolate syrup, omit or reduce the amount of sweetener.

- 1 cup cashew hemp milk
- 2 teaspoons cacao, chocolate powder or chocolate syrup
- 2 teaspoons xylitol
- ½ teaspoon lecithin
- ½ teaspoon tocotrienols
- ½ teaspoon chicory
- ¼ teaspoon vanilla extract

Blend well.

Cashew Hemp Orange Vanilla Milk

16 ounces

- 2 cups plain cashew hemp milk
- 1 ½ Tablespoons coconut palm sugar
- ½ teaspoon vanilla extract
- ½ teaspoon orange extract

Blend well.

Cashew Hemp Orange Vanilla Banana Smoothie

16 ounces

- 2 cups cashew hemp milk
- ½ cup banana, fresh or frozen
- 1 teaspoon orange juice
- 1 teaspoon coconut palm sugar
- ½ teaspoon orange zest

Blend well.

Lavender Honey Cashew Milk

16 ounces

Delicious over crushed ice.

- 2 cups filtered water
- ½ cup cashews
- 6 Tablespoons Lavender Honey Simple Syrup
    (see recipe below)

Blend well.
Strain.

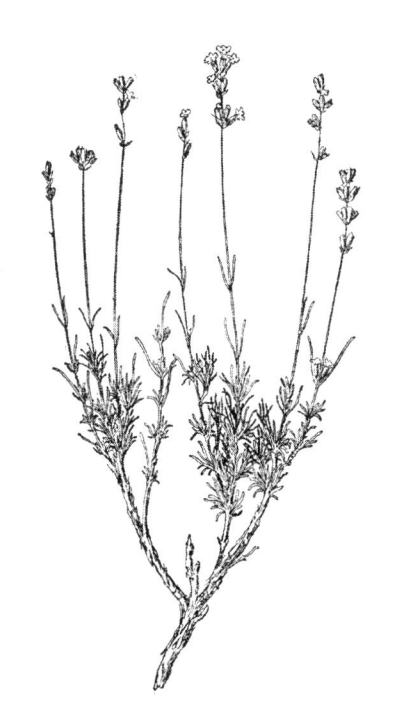

Lavender Honey Simple Syrup

- 1 ½ cups filtered water
- ⅓ cup raw honey
- 1 teaspoon dried lavender
- 3–4 fresh English Lavender blossoms

Gently heat water and honey until the honey dissolves.
Add lavender.
Turn off the heat and let steep for about 5 minutes.
Cool and strain.
Store in a glass jar in the refrigerator.
Use 3 Tablespoons of Lavender Honey syrup to 1 cup of nut milk.

Lavender Honey Ginger Sparkling Cashew Milk
16 ounces

- 8 ounces lavender honey cashew milk
- 8 ounces sparkling water
- 1 teaspoon candied ginger, or to taste

Blend the lavender honey cashew milk and ginger.
Add the sparkling water.
Serve in a tall glass with ice.

Cashew Pomegranate Orange Milk
12 ounces

- 1 cup plain cashew milk
- ½ cup pomegranate seeds
- ½ cup orange juice
- ⅛ teaspoon stevia

Blend well.
Strain.

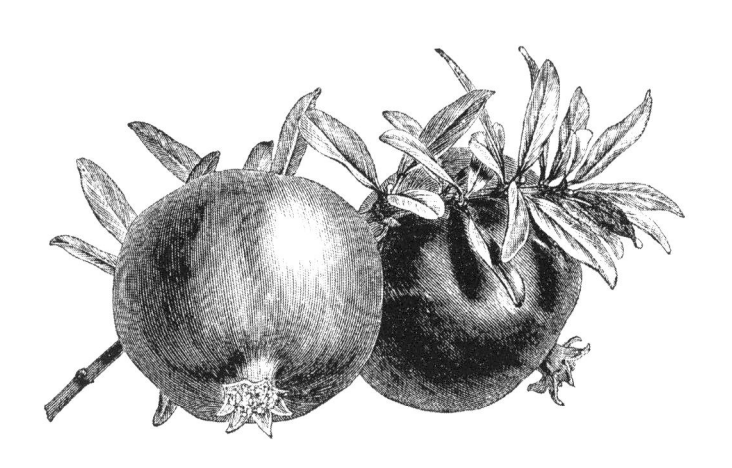

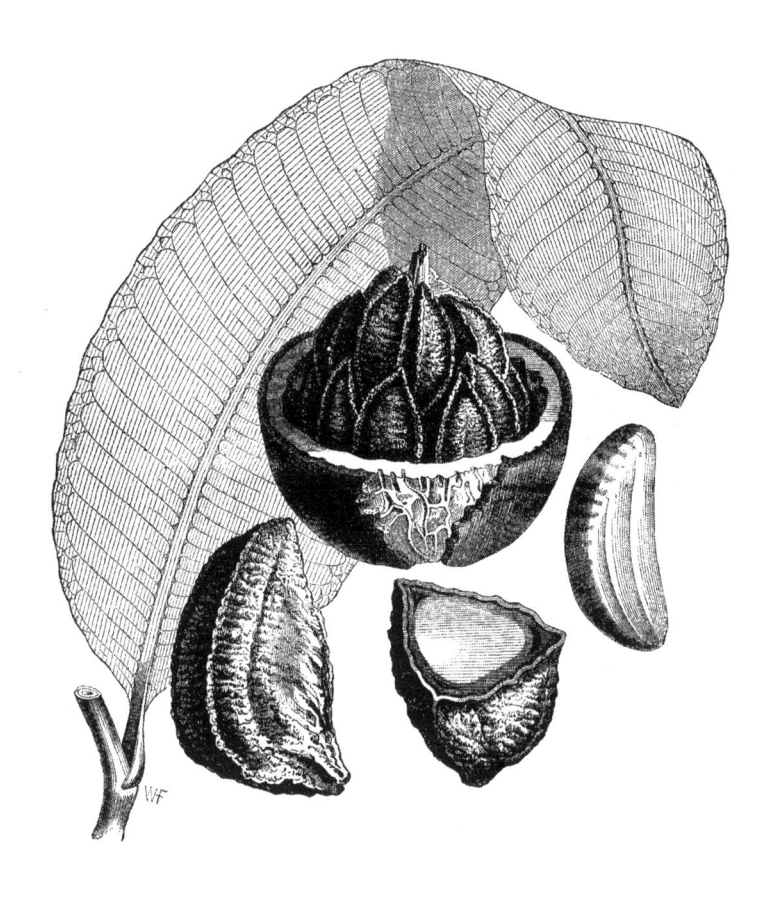

Brazil Nuts

Brazil nuts have a very unique and distinctive flavor. The seed is from the fruit of the Bertholletia tree, which is native to South America, primarily found in the Brazilian Amazon. The trees are well known for their towering height of over 160 feet and, most interestingly, are wild harvested and not grown on plantations.

Brazil nuts are extremely nutrient-rich, containing (by weight) approximately 18% protein, along with many minerals, including copper, niacin, magnesium, vitamin E and a high amount of selenium.

Because brazil nuts are high in fats, about 65% by weight, I always store them in the refrigerator.

> Brazil Nuts Do Not Require Soaking

Simple Brazil Nut Milk
16 ounces

- 2   cups water
- ½   cup brazil nuts

Blend well.
Strain.

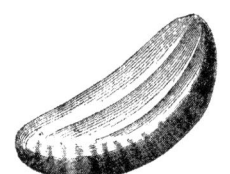

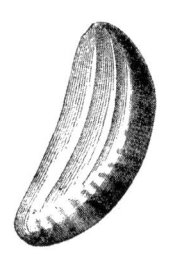

Creamy Brazil Nut Milk
One quart

This recipe uses fewer brazil nuts and produces a mild flavored milk. The addition of tocotrienols (tocos), lecithin and chicory add body and increase the nutritional profile.

- 4   cups water
- ½   cup brazil nuts
- 4   Tablespoons chicory
- 3   Tablespoons tocotrienols
- 2   Tablespoons lecithin

Blend the water and brazil nuts.
Strain.
Pour the milk back into a clean blender.
Add tocos, lecithin and chicory.
Blend well.

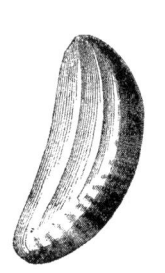

Creamy Brazil Praline Smoothie
Single 8 ounce serving

    1   cup creamy brazil nut milk
    ¾   cup "Almond Dream Praline Crunch" frozen dessert*
    ½   cup banana, fresh or frozen

Blend well.

* You will find this in the frozen section of your health food store.

Brazil Almond Milk
16 ounces

    1   cup brazil nut milk, plain or creamy
    1   cup almond milk

Blend.

Brazil Almond Goji Berry Milk
Single 8 ounce serving

You will have delightful bits of goji berries in your milk!

    1   cup filtered water
    ¼   cup almonds
    5-7 brazil nuts
    2   Tablespoons goji berries
    ½   teaspoon raw honey

Blend the water, almonds and brazil nuts.
Strain.
Pour the milk back into a clean blender.
Add goji berries and honey.
Blend well.

Brazil Almond Chocolate Mint Milk

Single 8 ounce serving

- ½ cup brazil nut milk, plain or creamy
- ½ cup almond milk
- 1 ½ Tablespoons Chocolate Mint Hazelnut Rawtella*
- 1 teaspoon coconut palm sugar

Blend well.
Pour over crushed ice.

*Rawtella can be found at your local health food store, or online. They have several delicious flavors!

You can substitute chocolate syrup, approximately 1 Tablespoon.

If the syrup is sweetened, omit the coconut palm sugar.

Peach Banana Brazil Nut Smoothie

Single 8 ounce serving

- 1 cup brazil nut milk
- ½ cup fresh, sweet, seasonal peaches
- ⅓ cup banana, fresh or frozen
- 1 teaspoon raw honey

Blend well.

Raspberry Coconut Anise Brazil Nut Smoothie

Single 8 ounce serving

- 1 cup brazil nut milk
- 1 Tablespoon coconut milk
- ½ cup raspberries, fresh or frozen
- ½ teaspoon raw honey
- ¼ teaspoon anise seed
- dash of stevia

Blend well.

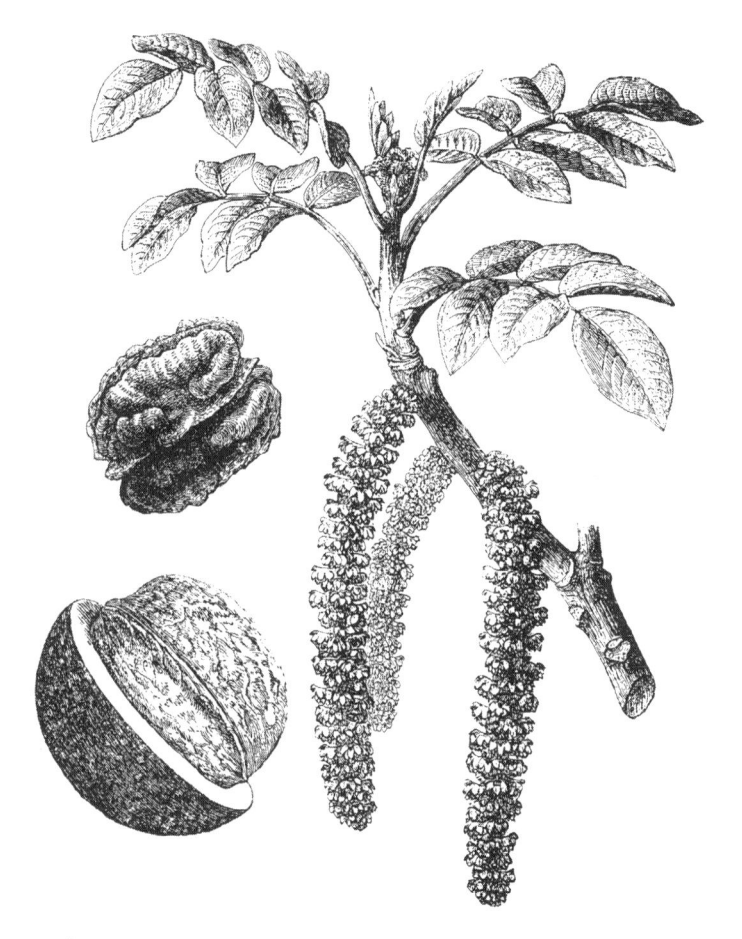

Walnuts

The worldwide production of walnuts comes from China, the United States, Iran, Turkey, the Ukraine, Mexico, Romania, India, France and Chile.

The United States is the world's largest exporter of walnuts, and the Sacramento and San Joaquin valleys of California produce over 90% of commercial English walnuts.

When it comes to walnuts, nearly two decades of research at renowned universities worldwide have shown walnuts to be a high density source of nutrients, including proteins and essential fatty acids.

Walnuts are unique compared to other nuts because they are predominantly composed of polyunsaturated fatty acids and are the only nut that contain a significant amount of alpha-linoleic acid (ALA), the plant-based source of omega-3 fatty acids.

I have found that walnuts can become rancid quickly, so for that reason, I always store them in the refrigerator or a very cool, dry and dark location.

If the nuts are not fresh, the flavor of the milk will not be the best.

I love the flavor of freshly made walnut milk, plain without sweeteners. However, the ratio of water to nuts is important, as using too many walnuts will produce a bitter milk.

Walnut Soak Time:
approximately 4 hours

Discard soak water

Simple Walnut Milk

16 ounces

For a change of pace, use walnut milk over granola, cereal or oatmeal.

- 2 cups filtered water
- ½ cup walnuts

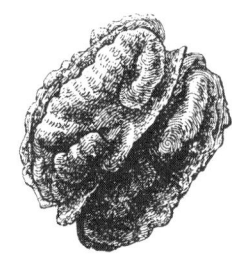

Blend well.
Strain.

Walnut Date Milk

16 ounces

This is just so darn good!

Medjool dates come in many sizes. I like to purchase the medium to large dates. They are soft and creamy and will easily emulsify in the milk.

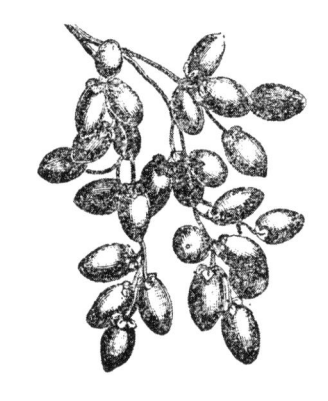

- 2 cups filtered water
- ½ cup walnuts
- 2 medjool dates, medium/large, pitted

Blend well.
Strain.

OPTIONAL:

If you prefer to have the date pieces in your milk as opposed to a smooth texture:

Make the walnut milk.
Strain.
Pour the walnut milk back into a clean blender.
Add the dates.
Blend well.

Creamy Walnut Coconut Milk

16 ounces

This makes a wonderful base for custard.

- 2 cups walnut date milk
- 1 ½ Tablespoons coconut milk
- 2 teaspoons lecithin

Blend well.

Creamy Walnut Coconut Cinnamon & Honey Milk

Single 8 ounce serving

- 1 cup walnut date milk
- 1 ½ teaspoons coconut milk
- 1 teaspoon lecithin
- ½ teaspoon raw honey, or to taste
- Dash of cinnamon

Blend well.

Walnut Almond Milk

16 ounces

- 2 cups filtered water
- ⅓ cup walnuts
- ⅓ cup almonds

Blend.
Strain.

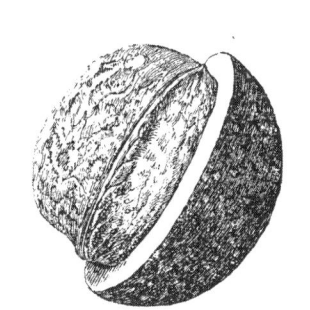

Walnut Almond Raisin Milk

Single 8 ounce serving

- 1 cup walnut almond milk
- 1 Tablespoon raisins
- 1 teaspoon maple syrup

Blend.
Strain.

OPTIONAL:
If you prefer to have raisin pieces in your milk as opposed to a smooth texture:

Make the walnut almond milk.
Strain.
Pour the milk back into a clean blender.
Add the raisins and maple syrup.
Blend well.

Walnut Almond Fall Smoothie

Single 8 ounce serving

This recipe will produce a smoothie with delightful bits of the figs, dates and cranberries!

- 1 cup walnut almond milk
- ⅓ cup fresh, ripe figs*
- 1 medjool date, medium/large, pitted
- 1 Tablespoon dried cranberries
- ⅓ cup banana, fresh or frozen (optional)

Blend well.
* Can substitute ¼ cup dried figs

Walnut Almond Anise Milk

Single 8 ounce serving

If you love the flavor of anise, give this one a try!

Makes a wonderful base for a dessert.

- 1 cup walnut almond milk
- ¾ teaspoon anise
- ¾ teaspoon xylitol

Blend well.
Strain, to sift out the anise.

Walnut Almond Anise Orange Milk

Single 8 ounce serving

This will delight your guests.

- 1 cup walnut almond anise milk
- 2 Tablespoons orange juice
- ¼ teaspoon orange zest
- Pinch of stevia

Blend well.
Serve over crushed ice.

Walnut Oat Milk

16 ounces

I use organic, raw (uncooked) rolled oats. The oats add body to the milk, however adding too much will make the milk chalky.

Try this over cooked oatmeal or as a smoothie base.

- 2 cups filtered water
- ½ cup walnuts
- ¼ cup organic rolled oats
- 1 teaspoon tocotrienols
- 1 teaspoon lecithin
- 1 teaspoon chicory

Blend water, walnuts and oats.
Strain.
Pour walnut oat milk back into a clean blender.
Add tocos, lecithin and chicory.
Blend well.

Walnut Oat Raisin Milk

16 ounces

This recipe will give you delicious raisin bits in your milk!

- 2 cups walnut oat milk
- 2 Tablespoons raisins
- 1 Tablespoon maple syrup
- ⅛ teaspoon cinnamon

Blend well.

Walnut Oat Raisin Banana Smoothie

16 ounces

- 2 cups walnut oat raisin milk
- 1 cup banana, fresh or frozen

Blend well.

Walnut Pear Milk

16 ounces

Simple, delicious flavors!

    2   cups pear juice
    ½   cup walnuts

Blend well.
Strain.

Walnut Pear Pomegranate Milk

Single 8 ounce serving

Don't miss this one!

    1   cup pear juice
    ¼   cup walnuts
    ⅓   cup pomegranate seeds

Blend well.
Strain.

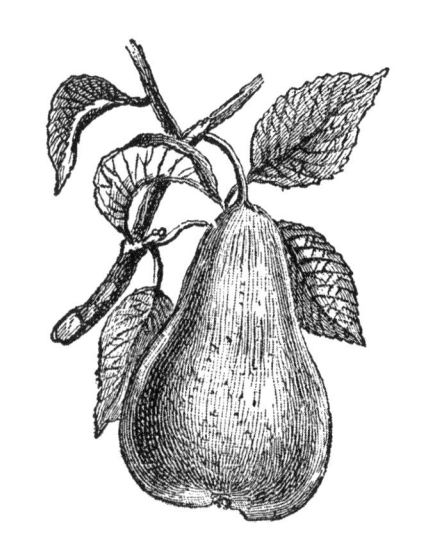

Walnut Pear Pomegranate Milk & Greens

Single 8 ounce serving

    1   cup pear juice
    ¼   cup walnuts
    ⅓   cup pomegranate seeds
    ¼   cup kale
    ¼   4" by 4" container of wheatgrass*

Blend well.
Strain.

*For Wheatgrass Tips see page 39.

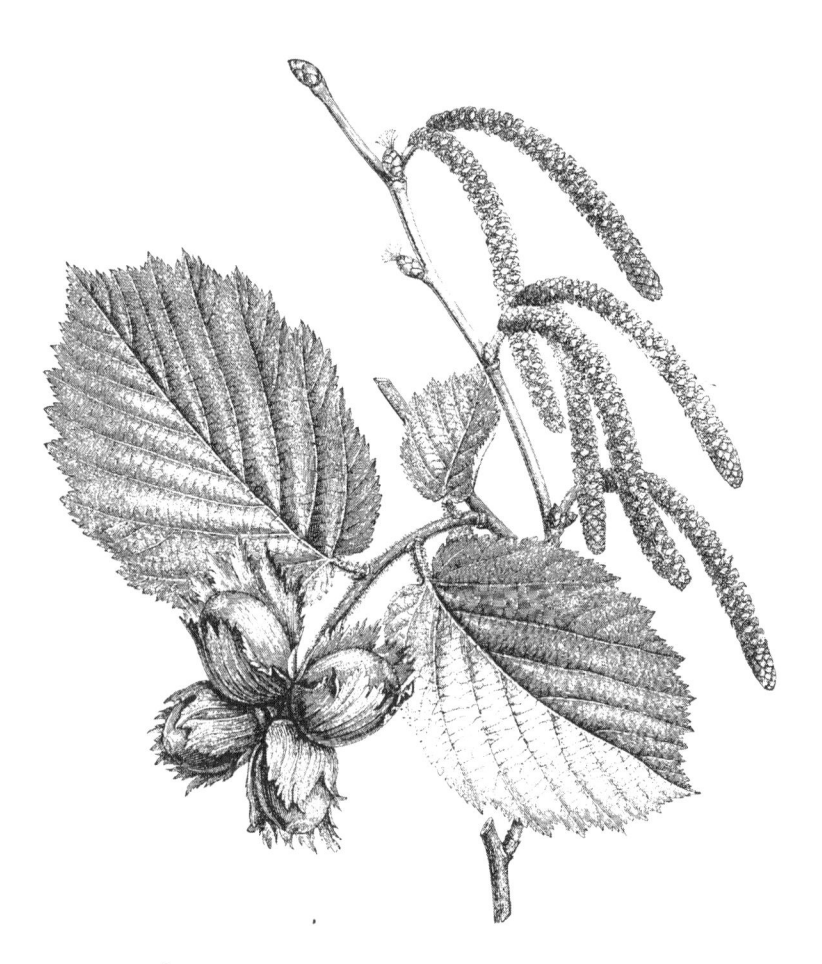

Hazelnut

Hazelnuts, also known as filberts, are grown in Turkey, Italy, Greece, Georgia, Spain, the UK and the US, with Turkey being the largest producer of hazelnuts in the world. In the US, 90% of the hazelnuts are grown in the rich soil of the Willamette Valley in Oregon and Washington.

I love the flavor of hazelnuts and they are one of the few nuts that I often roast to bring out the distinctive hazelnut flavor. I purchase unflavored, raw hazelnuts and soak them before roasting or dehydrating.

Hazelnuts are rich in protein, complex carbohydrates, dietary fiber, iron, calcium and vitamin E.

> ## Hazelnut Soak Time:
> approximately 6 to 8 hours
>
> Discard soak water

ROASTING HAZELNUTS (OPTIONAL):

After soaking, roast at 250 degrees F. for about 35 minutes, or dehydrate at approximately 110 to 115 degrees F. for up to 24 hours.

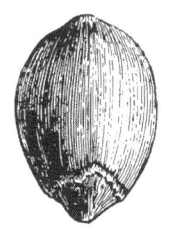

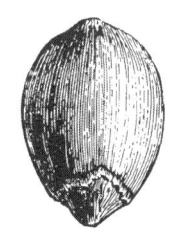

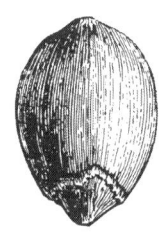

Simple Hazelnut Milk
16 ounces

- 2 cups filtered water
- ¾ cup hazelnuts

Blend.
Strain.

Creamy Hazelnut Milk
16 ounces

- 2 cups filtered water
- ¾ cup hazelnuts
- 1 Tablespoon chicory
- 1 Tablespoon tocotrienols
- 1 ½ teaspoons lecithin

Blend water and hazelnuts.
Strain.
Pour milk back into a clean blender.
Add chicory, tocos and lecithin.
Blend well.

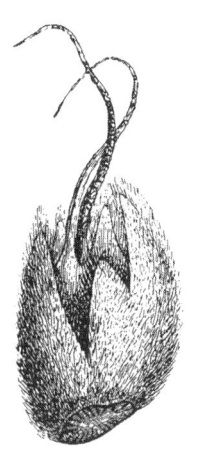

Sweetened Hazelnut Milk
16 ounces

- 2 cups filtered water
- ¾ cup hazelnuts
- 1 Tablespoon chicory
- 1 Tablespoon tocotrienols
- 1 ½ teaspoons lecithin
- 1 ½ teaspoons light agave

Blend water and hazelnuts.
Strain.
Pour the milk back into a clean blender.
Add chicory, tocos, lecithin and agave.
Blend well.

Chocolate Hazelnut Milk

Single 8 ounce serving

- 1 cup hazelnut milk, simple or creamy
- 1 Tablespoon cacao or chocolate powder
- 1 ½ teaspoons agave nectar

Blend well.

Hot Chocolate Hazelnut Milk

Place chocolate hazelnut milk in frother or gently heat on the stove.

Hazelnut Orange Date Milk

Single 8 ounce serving

- 1 cup hazelnut milk, simple or creamy
- 1 ½ Tablespoons unsweetened, organic, frozen orange juice concentrate
- 1 medjool date, medium/large, pitted

Blend well.

Hazelnut Orange Raspberry Smoothie

Single 10 ounce serving

- 10 ounces hazelnut milk, simple or creamy
- 2 Tablespoons unsweetened, organic, frozen orange juice concentrate
- 2 medjool dates, medium/large, pitted
- ½ cup frozen bananas
- ⅓ cup raspberries, fresh or frozen

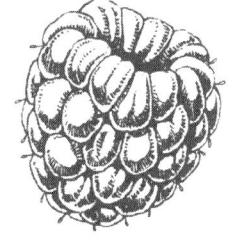

Blend well.

Hazelnut Banana Cinnamon Smoothie
Single 8 ounce serving

    1   cup hazelnut milk, simple or creamy
    ½   cup banana, fresh or frozen
    2   teaspoons raw honey
    ¼   teaspoon cinnamon

Blend well.

Hazel Brazil Nut Milk
16 ounces

Delicious without any sweetener!

    ½   cup hazelnuts
    ⅓   cup brazil nuts

Blend well.
Strain.

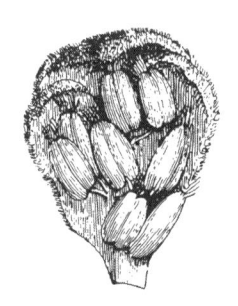

Hazel Brazil Nut Chocolate Milk
Single 8 ounce serving

    1   cup hazel brazil nut milk
    1   Tablespoon chocolate syrup*

Blend well.

*Chocolate syrups are usually sweetened, so taste before you add sweetener.

If you use cocoa or cacao powder add 2 teaspoons of light agave.

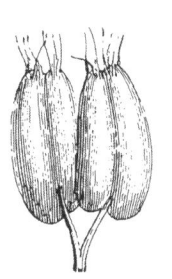

Hazel Brazil Nut Decadence

Single 8 ounce serving

You must give this a try!

- 1 cup hazel brazil nut milk
- 1 Tablespoon chocolate syrup
- 1 Tablespoon Rawtella Silk*

*You can find Rawtella in your health food store or online. This recipe calls for the "Silk" blend, which is a white chocolate hazelnut spread.

Rawtella and chocolate syrup are sweetened, so no additional sweetener is necessary.

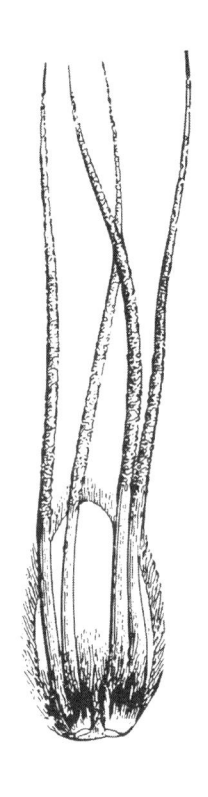

Blend well.

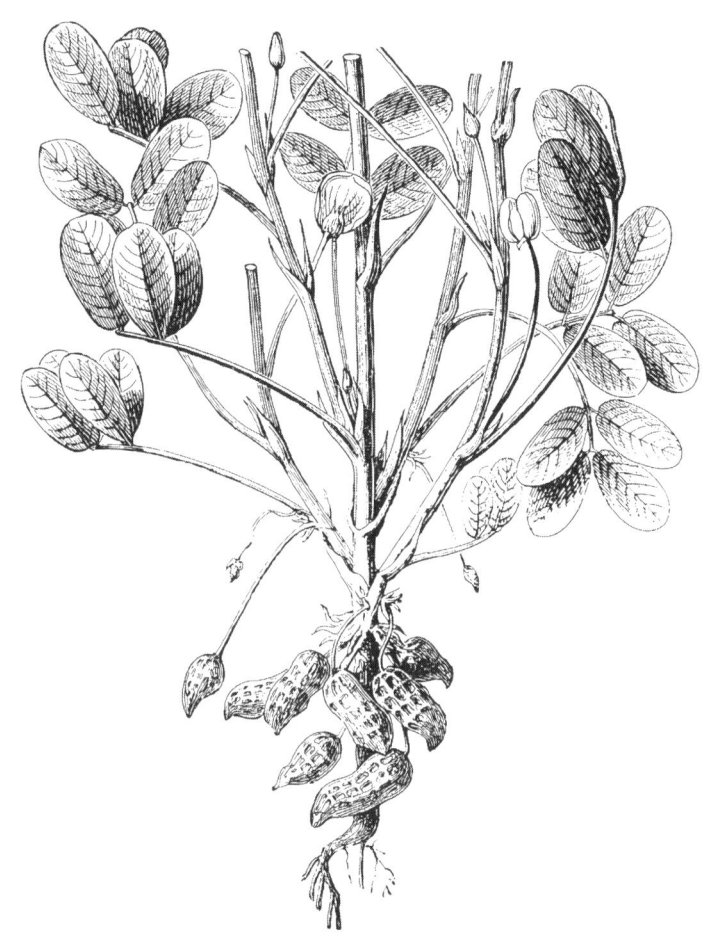

Peanuts

A though called a nut, the peanut is a legume and part of the pea and bean family.

Archeologists have dated the oldest specimens to about 7,600 years, found in Peru with cultivation spreading as far as Mesoamerica and later spread worldwide by European traders.

These legumes grow in warm climates on a flowering plant with the peanut developing underground. The light, porous shell of the peanut allows the nut to easily absorb materials leached from the soil. Peanuts that are grown conventionally are treated with a high level of pesticides, so it's important to buy organic peanut products and to refrigerate your peanut butter to prevent fungal growth.

China leads in the production of peanuts, with approximately 41% of overall world production, followed by India, which produces approximately 18%, and the United States with approximately 6.8%.

Peanuts are high in protein, vitamins and minerals, including vitamin E, niacin, folic acid, calcium, copper, zinc, potassium, iron and magnesium.

> ### Peanut Soak Time:
> approximately 6 to 8 hours
> Make sure you are soaking raw (unroasted) peanuts
> Discard soak water

I love the flavor of lightly roasted organic peanuts.

ROASTING PEANUTS (OPTIONAL):

After soaking, roast at 250 degrees F. for about 35 minutes, or dehydrate at approximately 110 to 115 degrees F. for up to 24 hours.

Simple Peanut Milk
16 ounces

- 2 cups filtered water
- ⅔ cups peanuts, raw or roasted

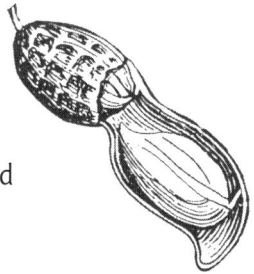

Blend well.
Strain.

Sweetened Peanut Milk

16 ounces

- 2 cups filtered water
- ⅔ cup peanuts, raw or roasted
- 1 Tablespoon coconut palm sugar

Blend well.
Strain.

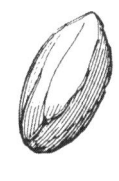

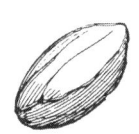

Peanut Grape Milk

Single 8 ounce serving

This tastes like peanut butter & jelly!

- 1 cup filtered water
- ⅓ cup peanuts, raw or roasted
- 2 Tablespoons unsweetened, organic grape juice concentrate
- ½ teaspoon lecithin
- ½ teaspoon tocotrienols
- ½ teaspoon chicory powder

Blend water, peanuts and grape concentrate.
Strain.
Pour milk back into a clean blender.
Add lecithin, tocos and chicory.
Blend well.

Peanut Banana Honey Smoothie

Single 8 ounce serving

- 1 cup unsweetened peanut milk
- ½ Tablespoon raw honey
- ⅓ cup banana, fresh or frozen

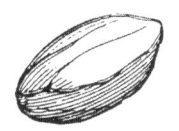

Blend well.

Peanut Chocolate Milk

Single 8 ounce serving

    1   cup unsweetened peanut milk
    1 ½ teaspoons cacao powder
    1   teaspoon agave
    ¼   teaspoon vanilla

Blend well.

Peanut Chocolate Malt Banana Smoothie

Single 8 ounce serving

    1   cup unsweetened peanut milk
    ⅓   cup banana, fresh or frozen
    1 ½ teaspoons cacao powder
    1   teaspoon agave
    ½   teaspoon mesquite powder
    ½   teaspoon maca powder
    ¼   teaspoon vanilla

Blend well.

Peanut Sesame Milk

Single 8 ounce serving

    1   cup unsweetened peanut milk
    2   Tablespoons sesame seeds, raw or slightly toasted
    1   teaspoon honey

Blend well. Strain.

Peanut Sesame Chocolate Banana Smoothie

Single 8 ounce serving

    1   cup sesame peanut milk
    ⅓   cup banana, fresh or frozen
    1   Tablespoon chocolate syrup

Blend well.

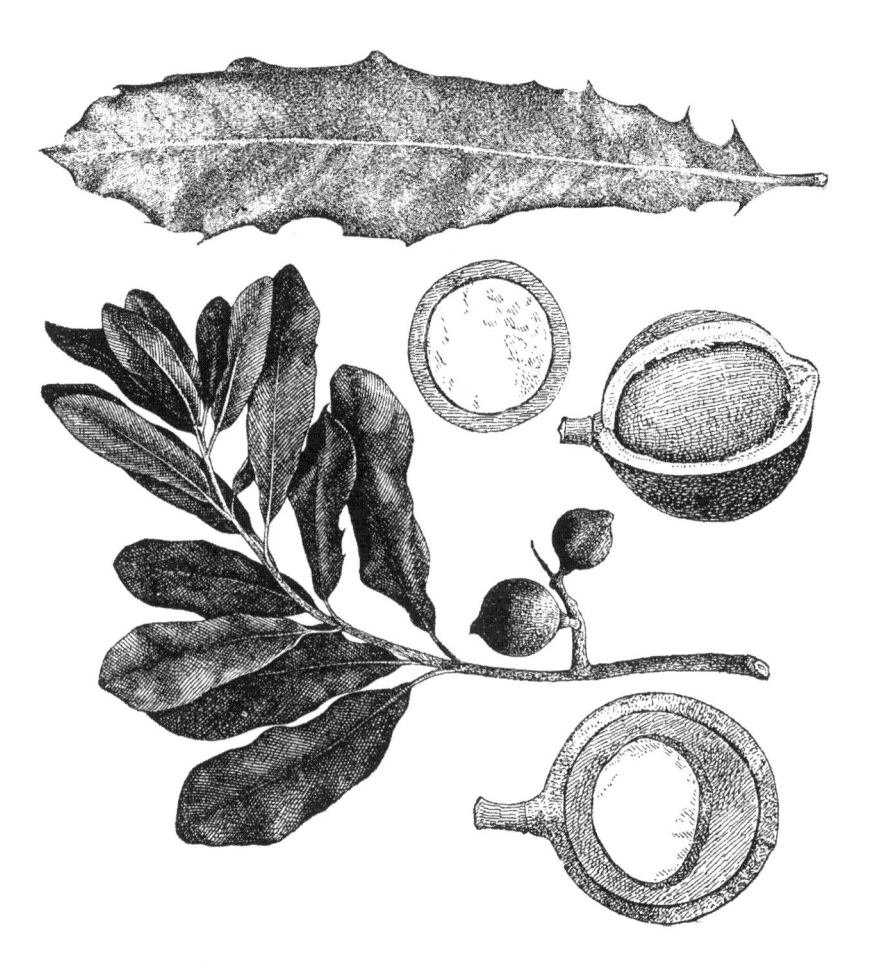

Macadamia Nuts

Macadamia nuts were a small boutique industry in Australia during the late 19th and early 20th centuries and, in the 1920s, became extensively planted as a commercial crop in Hawaii.

Outside of Hawaii and Australia, macadamia nuts are also commercially produced in South Africa, Brazil, California, Costa Rica, Israel, Kenya, Bolivia, New Zealand, Colombia, Guatemala and Malawi, with Australia as the world's largest commercial producer.

Compared to other nuts and seeds, macadamia nuts are high in fat and low in protein with the highest amount of monounsaturated fats of any nut. Because of the high fat content, I recommend that you keep them refrigerated.

Macadamia nuts make delicious milk and due to their high cost and high fat content, I use macadamia's as a treat. You will find a recipe in the cashew section for a "vegan nog" that combines cashews and macadamias. Definitely give that recipe a try!

I love macadamia nuts raw, lightly roasted, roasted & salted and covered with chocolate!

Macadamia nut milk is deliciously rich and makes great custard!

> Macadamia Nuts Do Not Require Soaking

Simple Macadamia Nut Milk
Single 8 ounce serving

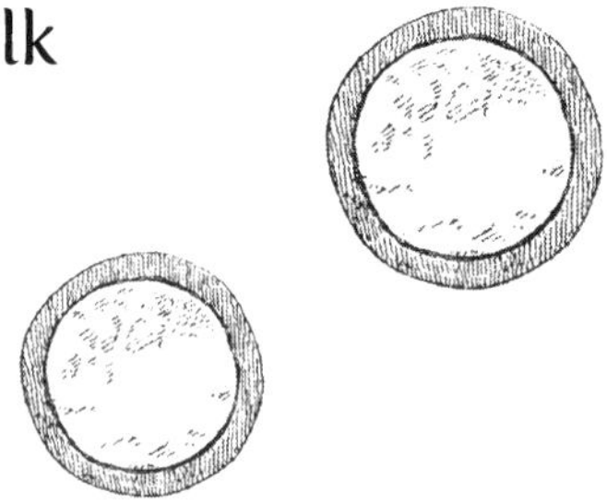

- 1 cup filtered water
- ⅓ cup macadamia nuts

Blend well.
Strain.

Sweetened Macadamia Nut Milk
Single 8 ounce serving

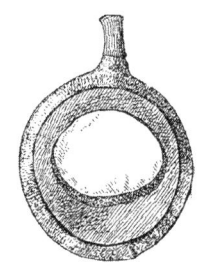

- 1 cup filtered water
- ⅓ cup macadamia nuts
- 1 teaspoon xylitol

Blend well.
Strain.

Macadamia Coconut Milk

Single 7 ounce serving

- ½ cup filtered water or coconut water
- ⅓ cup coconut milk
- ¼ cup macadamia nuts
- 2 teaspoons coconut palm sugar

Blend well.
Strain.

Macadamia Banana Coconut Smoothie

14 ounce serving

- 1 cup filtered water or coconut water
- ½ cup macadamia nuts
- ⅔ cup coconut milk
- ⅔ cup banana, fresh or frozen
- 1 ½ Tablespoons coconut palm sugar

Blend water and macadamia nuts.
Strain.
Pour milk back into a clean blender.
Add coconut milk, banana and coconut palm sugar.
Blend well.

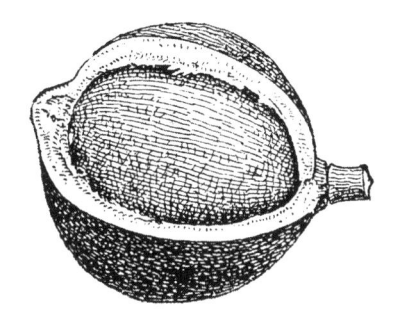

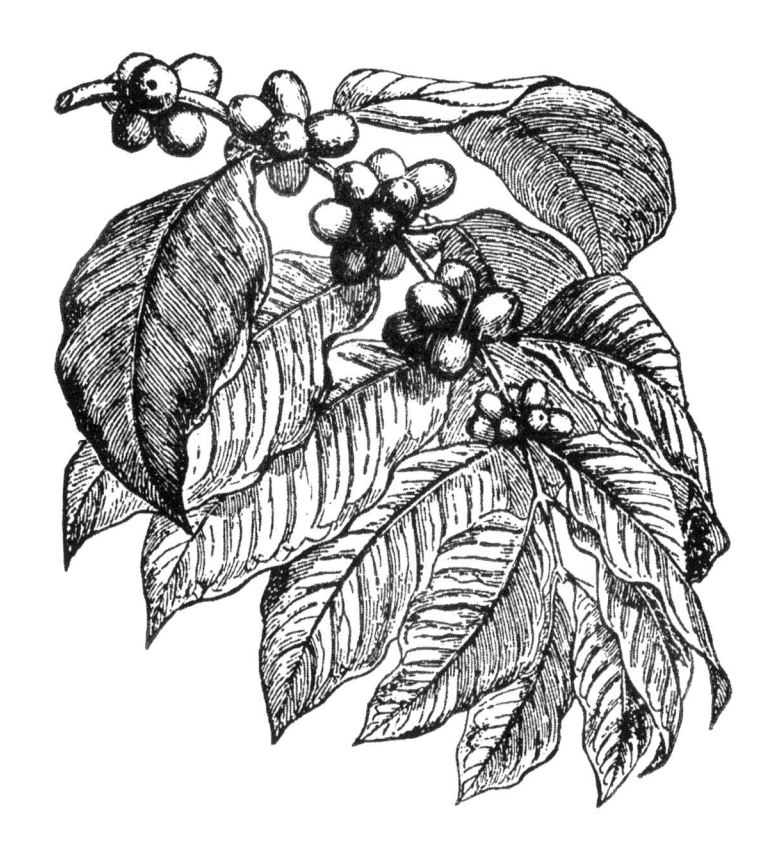

Coffee & Nut Milk

Almond and hazelnut milks are my favorite choices for coffee and coffee substitutes. To bring out the fullest flavor when using these nuts for coffee, I roast them. However, whether raw or roasted, almonds and hazelnuts make a great pairing with coffee.

FOR ROASTING (OPTIONAL):

After soaking, roast at 250 degrees F. for about 35 minutes, or dehydrate at approximately 110 to 115 degrees F. for up to 24 hours.

> **KEEP IN MIND:**
>
> - When preparing nut milk specifically for coffee or when frothing for lattes, you'll get the best flavor by using a higher ratio of nuts to water than a general nut milk recipe.
> - If your nut milk has high water content, flavors will be diluted.
> - If your coffee is very hot, nut milk may curdle.

Frothing Nut Milk

Frothing nut milk does not produce the same results as dairy milk. Foam density is the combination of fats and proteins, and the particular composition of dairy milk protein has the ability to produce a very dense foam.

Unsweetened almond or hazelnut milk, with an approximate ratio of ¾ to 1 cup of nuts to 2 cups of water, foams well. It is best to foam plain, unsweetened milks.

Almond or Hazelnut Milk for Coffee and Lattes

16 ounces

This milk can be used for pouring into your coffee or you can froth it.

The strength of coffee is a personal taste. I love the flavor of coffee and my preference is at least half coffee and half nut milk. Experiment to find your favorite balance.

- 2 cups filtered water
- 1 cup almonds or hazelnuts, raw or roasted

Blend.
Strain.

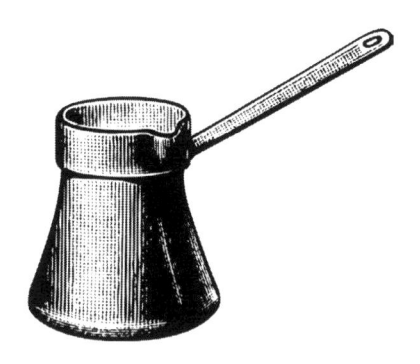

FOR COFFEE:
Add desired amount of milk. I recommend frothing the milk. Sweeten to taste.

FOR LATTES:
Use 1 ounce of espresso to 6 to 7 ounces of frothed milk. Adjust the balance to your preference. Sweeten to taste.

Iced Coffee with Almond or Hazelnut Milk
16 ounces

This method is prefered for making iced coffee. It is also excellent as a base for custards and other desserts.

Note: If the coffee has just been brewed, allow it to cool. It may be too hot to handle through the straining cloth.

    2   cups strong brewed coffee
    1   cup almonds or hazelnuts, raw or roasted
    Sweeten to taste

Place coffee, nuts and sweetener into blender.
Blend well.
Strain, then refrigerate.
To serve, pour over ice.

Coffee Substitutes

There are many coffee substitutes on the market. Our palates are unique and individual, so if you are looking for a coffee substitute, here are a few to try.

Cafix, Inka, Pero (dark roast), Roma, Rocamojo (soybeans), Teeccino (sweeter), Roastaroma, Raja Cup, Ayruvedic Roast.

Follow the product instructions to make your brew.

Sweeten to taste.

Add frothed almond or hazelnut milk.

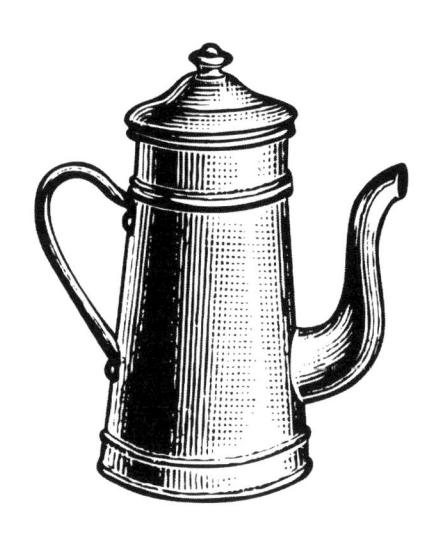

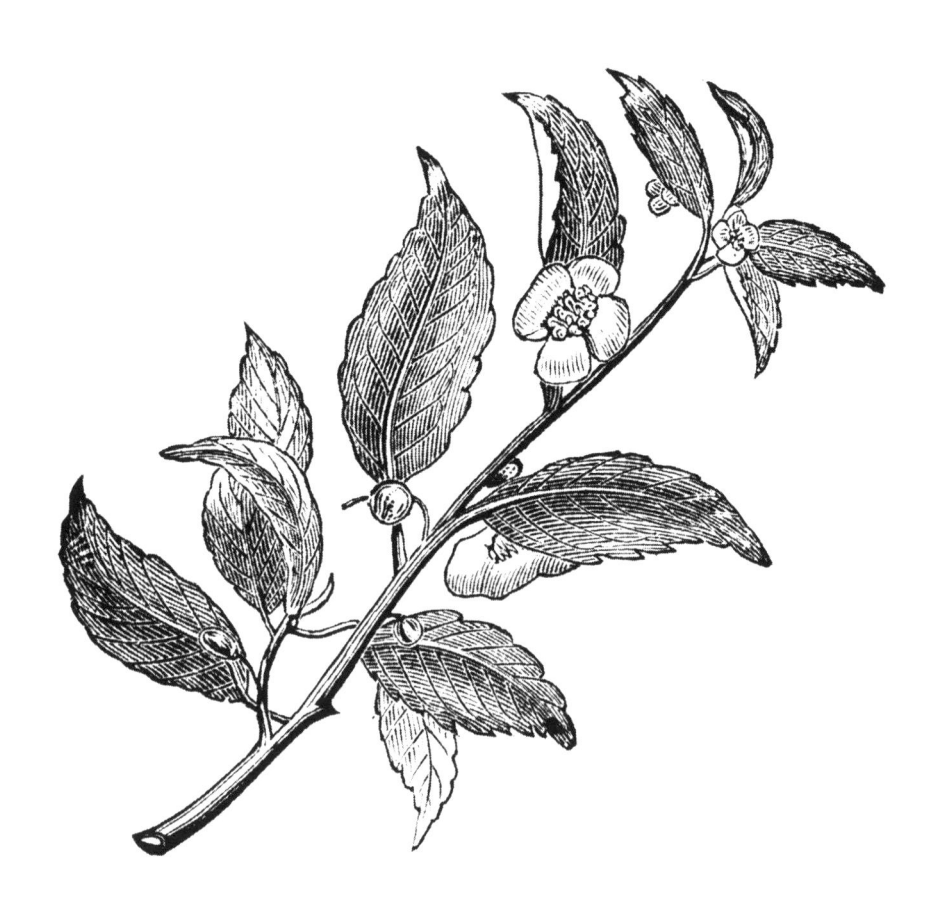

Teas & Nut Milk

Green, black or herbal—teas are a time-honored ritual!
Morning, afternoon or evening,
During, after or between meals,
Lingering over a cup of tea seems to hit the spot.

From artisanal shops that specialize in blending their own teas to the numerous flavors and brands on market shelves, choices abound—and I share some of my favorites with you.

TEA TIME?

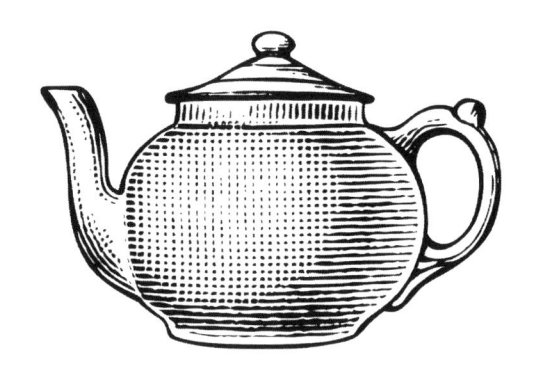

KEEP IN MIND:

- As with coffee, when using nut milk for tea, you'll get the best flavor by using a higher ratio of nuts to water than a general nut milk recipe. If your nut milk has high water content, flavors are diluted.

- I recommend a ratio of 1 ½ to 2 cups of almonds to 1 quart of water for a creamy almond milk.

- If the water used for tea is too hot, the nut milk may curdle.

- Experiment with the ratio of nut milk to tea; you may like less or more.

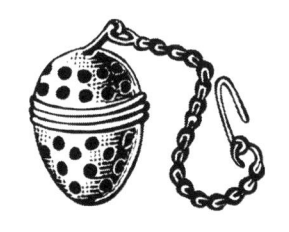

Chai

Recognized as a beverage from India made by brewing black tea and milk with a mixture of aromatic Indian spices and herbs.

Chai Tea & Almond Milk
Individual serving

Chai flavors vary greatly, so try different blends until you find one you like, or you can try your hand at making a mixture at home!

Brew a strong blend of your favorite chai tea

- 6 ounces chai tea
- 3 ounces almond milk

Brew your tea.
Place in tall glass.
Add milk. I recommend frothing the milk.
Sweeten to taste. I recommend coconut palm sugar.

Bengal Spice Tea & Almond Milk
Single serving

Bengal Spice is a caffeine free interpretation of Chai made by Celestial Seasonings and has great flavor.

- 1 tea bag Bengal Spice
- 5 ounces boiling water
- 3-4 ounces almond milk

Steep tea about 3 minutes.
Add milk. I recommend frothing the milk.
Sweeten to taste. I recommend coconut palm sugar.

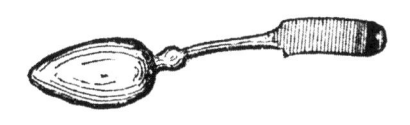

Rooibos Tea

You will find many blends of Rooibos, a Southern Africa tea, that is also known as bush tea, South African red tea, or red tea. Rooibos is becoming more popular in Western countries due to its high level of antioxidants, lack of caffeine, and low tannin levels.

Rooibos Tea & Almond Milk

Single serving

- 1 tea bag rooibos tea
- 6 ounces boiling water
- 3-4 ounces almond milk

Steep tea about 3 minutes.
Add milk. I recommend frothing the milk.
Sweeten to taste. I recommend coconut palm sugar or stevia.

Rooibos & Coconut Milk

Single serving

- 1-2 tea bags rooibos tea
- 6 ounces boiling water
- 1 ½ Tablespoons coconut milk

Steep tea about 3 minutes.
If you like a stronger flavor tea, use 2 tea bags.
Add coconut milk.
Sweeten to taste. I recommend coconut palm sugar, agave or stevia.

I recommend adding the tea, coconut milk and sweetener into a personal blender and mix well.

Matcha Green Tea

Matcha is premium green tea powder from Japan, used for tea or as an ingredient in recipes. While other green teas are grown throughout the world, matcha is unique to Japan. Matcha is renowned for its numerous health benefits, being rich in nutrients, antioxidants, fiber and chlorophyll.

Matcha Green Tea & Almond Milk
Single serving

- 6 ounces almond milk
- 1 teaspoon matcha powder

Add ingredients to frother using cold, warm or hot setting. If you don't have a frother, whisk until blended. Sweeten to taste. I recommend xylitol.

Matcha Green Tea with Hemp & Banana
Single serving

- 8 ounces almond milk
- 1 ½ teaspoons of matcha powder
- ¼ cup fresh banana
- 2 teaspoons hemp seeds
- 1 teaspoon xylitol

Add ingredients to personal blender. Blend well.

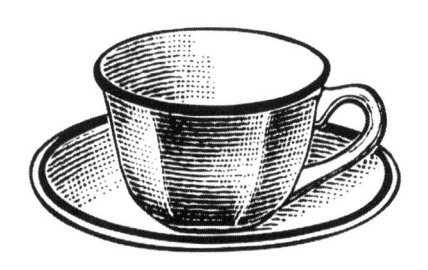

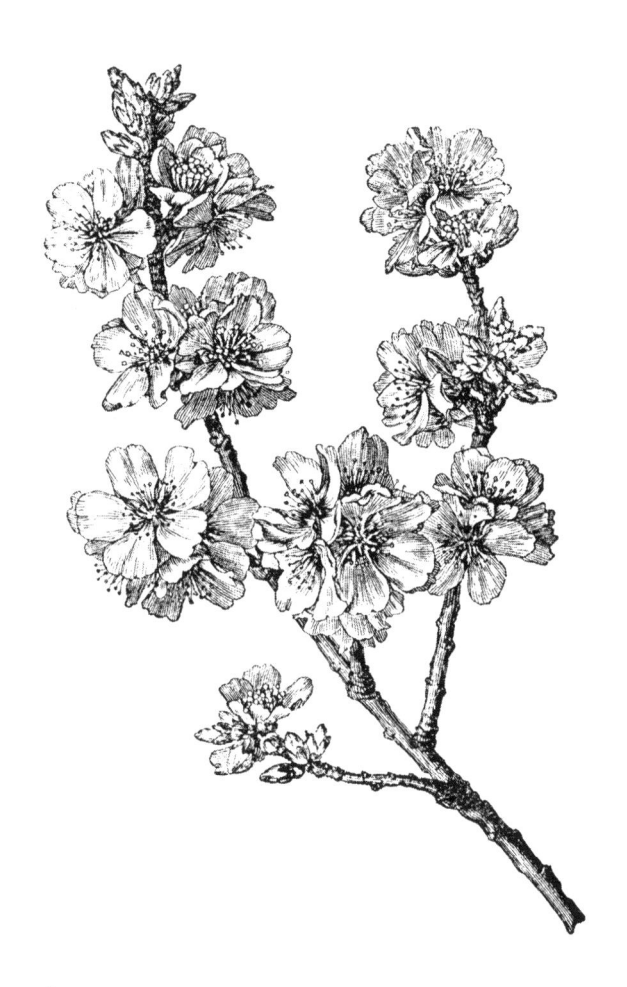

Soda Fountain Creams

Refreshing and delicous!

Growing up on the east coast, Saturday's ritual was going to our local soda shop and ordering an "egg cream," a soda fountain beverage that contained neither eggs nor cream. Egg creams are a wonderful childhood memory and although soda fountain shops are a thing of the past, this simple beverage made with milk, chocolate and carbonated water is a great treat for kids and adults!

> To prepare the base of almond milk for these soda fountain creams, I suggest using approximately 1 ¼ to 1 ½ cups of almonds to 1 quart of water.
>
> - I like to use Pellegrino for my soda fountain creams, however you can use any carbonated water.
> - It is best if all ingredients are cold.

Chocolate Soda Fountain Cream
Single 9 ounce serving

- 5 ounces almond milk
- 4 ounces pellegrino or other carbonated water
- 1 Tablespoon chocolate syrup, or to taste

Blend milk and chocolate syrup in a personal blender, or whisk vigorously in a tall glass.

Add carbonated water, stir and enjoy!

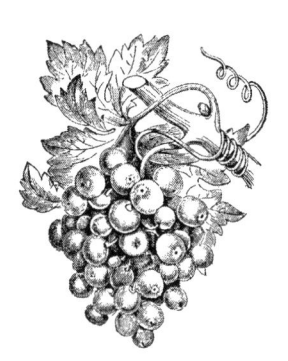

Grape Soda Fountain Cream
Single 8 ounce serving

- 5 ounces pellegrino or other carbonated water
- 3 ounces almond milk
- 1 ½ Tablespoons unsweetened, frozen grape juice concentrate

Blend milk and grape concentrate in a personal blender or whisk vigorously in a tall glass.

Add carbonated water, stir and enjoy!

Orange Soda Fountain Cream

Single 8 ounce serving

- 5 ounces pellegrino or other carbonated water
- 3 ounces almond milk
- 1 ½ Tablespoons unsweetened, frozen orange juice concentrate

Blend milk and orange concentrate in a personal blender or whisk vigorously in a tall glass.
Add carbonated water, stir and enjoy.

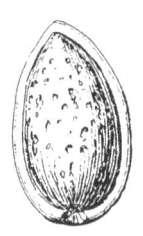

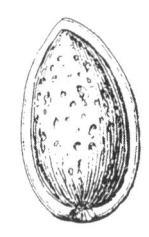

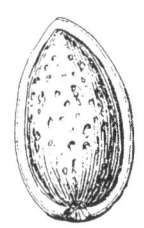

Milkshakes

Nut Milk Ice Cream Shakes
Tasty treats... and so easy to prepare!

A traditional milkshake consits of milk, ice cream and an optional flavoring.

The non-dairy ice cream market has been rapidly growing and I love all the delectable flavors available in our local health food stores. Companies are producing ice creams from coconut milk, rice milk, almond milk and even cashew milk.

SUGGESTIONS

In general, almond milk makes a great base for shakes. I recommend using one of the "light bodied" recipes that include tocotrienols (tocos) and lecithin.

I love Coconut Bliss ice cream and they have some great flavors! If you are using Coconut Bliss or another coconut milk ice cream, try using coconut milk as a base for your shake in place of almond milk.

When using a simple ice cream flavor like vanilla, you can add flavored syrups and concentrates of your choice such as strawberry, chocolate, amaretto and butter pecan, to name a few.

Basic Milkshake Recipe
Single serving

Best if the milk is cold
For a thicker shake, use more ice cream

- ⅓ cup cold nut milk of your choice
- 1 ¾ cups of your favorite non-dairy ice cream

Flavoring is optional, depending on the ice cream flavor you have chosen.

Blend well.

Visit our website at www.MilksAlive.com for a link to find natural organic syrups and concentrates made with low gyclemic sugars that are kosher, vegan and gluten free—and use your creativity!

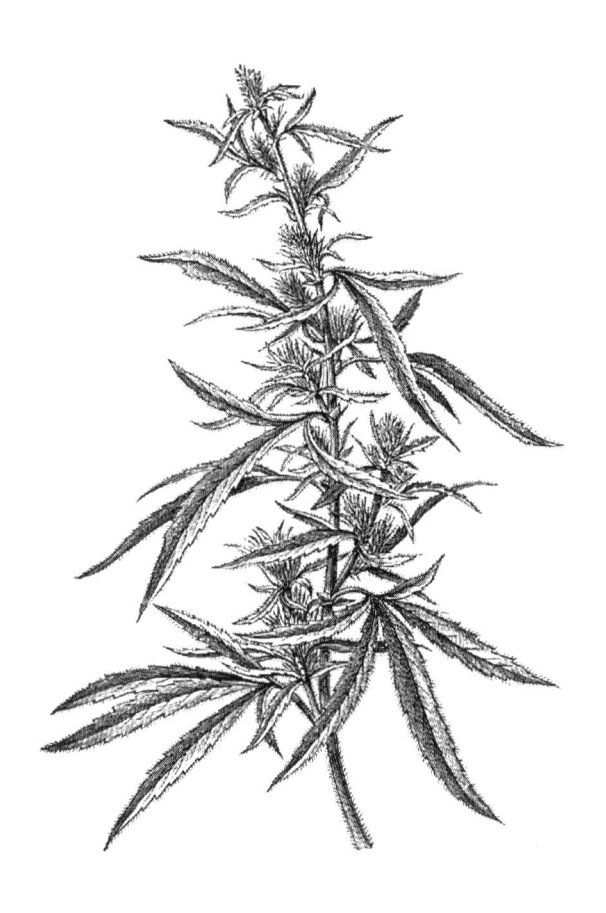

Hemp

Hemp is an extraordinary plant with a long and interesting history.

The hemp plant is often called nature's most perfect food, as the hemp seed provides a complete source of easily digestible protein, all eight essential amino acids and essential fatty acids. It has been used for producing clothing, paper, building materials and cosmetics.

Henry Ford built his first Motel T car from hemp! The engine was designed to run on hemp or other vegetable and seed fuels, and the plastic hemp panels were said to have an impact strength many times greater than steel.

The hemp plant produces 3 to 4 times more cellulose per acre than trees, the plants grow very quickly and there is no question that the production of hemp has substantialy less environmental impact than the production of oil.

All that being said, since 1937 it became illegal to grow industrial hemp in the United States, as the government does not make a distinction between industrial grade hemp and the commonly named hemp crop, marijuana. However, since 1998 the US has allowed the importation of food grade hemp.

FOR MAKING HEMP MILK, I SUGGEST:

- Use organic, shelled hemp seeds
- Strain the milk for a smooth texture
- Store seeds in the refrigerator or in freezer for long-term storage

> Hemp Seeds Do Not Require Soaking

Fresh hemp milk has a strong, nutty flavor and can have a bitter taste if you use too much.

Simple Hemp Milk
16 ounces

    2   cups filtered water
    ⅓   cup hemp seeds

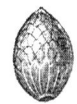

Blend well.
Strain.

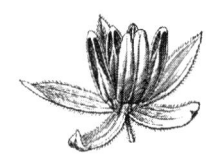

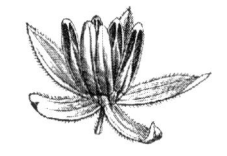

Sweetened Hemp Milk
16 ounces

- 2 cups filtered water
- ⅓ cup hemp seeds
- 1 Tablespoon coconut palm sugar
- 1 teaspoon tocotrienols
- 1 teaspoon lecithin

Blend hemp seeds and water.
Strain.
Pour milk back into a clean blender.
Add tocos, lecithin and coconut palm sugar.
Blend well.

Vanilla Hemp Milk
16 ounces

- 2 cups filtered water
- ⅓ cup hemp seeds
- 1 ½ Tablespoons coconut palm sugar
- 2 teaspoons tocotrienols
- 1 teaspoon lecithin
- ⅛ teasspoon vanilla bean

Blend water and hemp seeds.
Strain.
Pour milk back into a clean blender.
Add coconut palm sugar, tocos, lecithin and vanilla.
Blend well.

Hemp Milk with Coconut Water

Single 8 ounce serving

Simple and delicous!

- 1 cup coconut water
- 3 Tablespoons hemp seed

Blend well.
Strain.

Hemp Almond Milk with Coconut Water & Chia Seeds

Single 8 ounce serving

- 1 cup coconut water
- 3 Tablespoons hemp seeds
- 2 Tablespoons almonds
- 1 Tablespoon chia seeds
- Pinch of stevia

Blend coconut water, hemp seeds, almonds and stevia.
Strain.
Place milk into a mason jar and add chia seeds.
Shake vigorously and refrigerate.
Shake again in another 5 to 10 minutes.

Note: Chia seeds will clump at the bottom if not agitated when first added.

Hemp Cashew Milk

Single 8 ounce serving

- 1 cup filtered water
- 2 Tablespoons hemp seed
- 2 Tablespoons cashews

Blend well.
Strain.

Hemp Cashew Orange Date Milk
Single 8 ounce serving

- 1 cup filtered water
- 2 Tablespoons hemp seed
- 2 Tablespoons cashews
- 1 Tablespoon unsweetened, frozen orange juice concentrate
- 1 medjool date, medium/large, pitted

Blend water, hemp and cashews.
Strain.
Pour the milk back into a clean blender.
Add the orange concentrate and date.
Blend well.

Hemp Persimmon Smoothie
Single 8 ounce serving

If you'e a persimmon lover, as I am, the persimmon adds texture and flavor.

- 1 cup hemp milk, simple or sweetened
- ⅓ cup fresh, ripe persimmon

Blend well.

Hemp Persimmon Honey Cinnamon Smoothie
Single 8 ounce serving

- 1 cup unsweetened hemp milk
- ⅓ cup fresh ripe persimmon
- 1 teaspoon raw honey
- Pinch of cinnamon

Blend well.

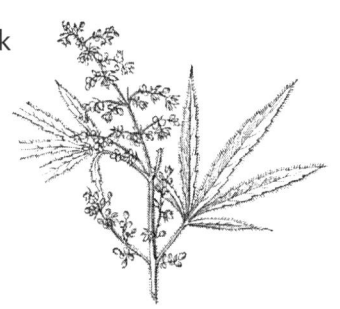

Hemp Pomegranate Coconut Banana Smoothie

Single 8 ounce serving

1	cup filtered water
½	cup pomegranate seeds
¼	cup banana, fresh or frozen
2	Tablespoons hemp seeds
1	Tablespoon coconut milk
1	teaspoon coconut palm sugar
1	teaspoon lecithin
1	teaspoon tocotrienols

Blend water, hemp and pomegranate seeds.
Strain.
Pour milk back into a clean blender.
Add coconut milk, coconut palm sugar, banana, lecithin and tocos.
Blend well.

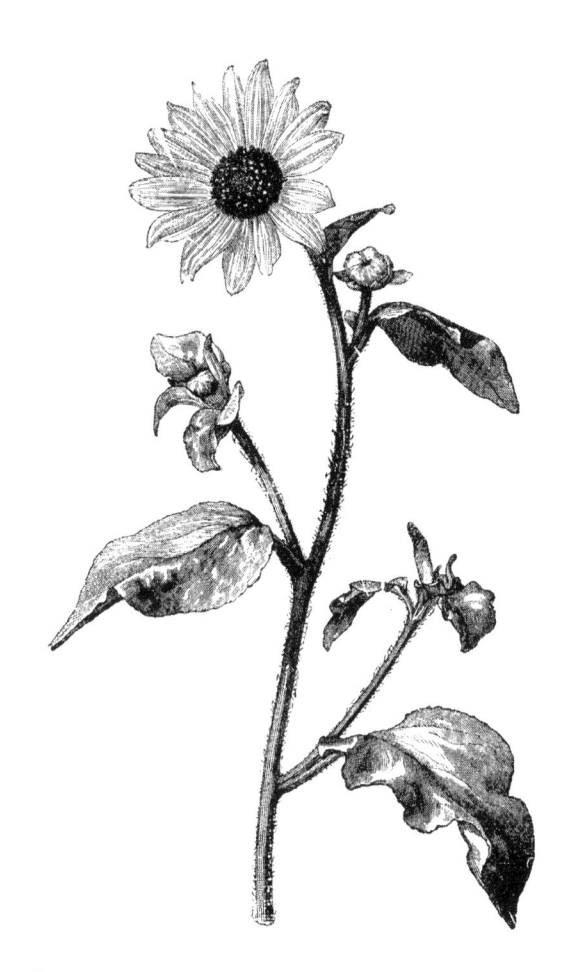

Sunflower Seeds

The sunflower is truly a gift of beauty.

One summer traveling through the south of France, we unexpectedly came upon acres of sunflowers in full bloom! What a breathtaking moment to be surrounded by these stunning flowers, enveloped in a sea of bright golden colors against the setting sun.

Sunflower seeds have been an important food and oil source for thousands of years. The seeds have a very high oil content with sunflower oil being one of the most popular oils in the world. Today, leading commercial producers include Russia, Peru, Argentina, Spain, France and China.

Sunflower seeds provide minerals, vitamin E, several B vitamins including thiamine and folic acid, dietary fiber, essential fatty acids and some amino acids, including tryptophan. Tryptophan is one of the building blocks of DNA and vital to the production of serotonin and melatonin.

After soaking, sunflower seeds have a milder flavor and they still maintain a crunch. I soak enough seeds for making milk with some left over to roast or dehydrate for garnishes on anything from soups to salads.

Sunflower Soak Time:
approximately 10 to 12 hours

If you soak them longer, I recommend rinsing and changing the water about halfway through the process.

Moist, soaked seeds will quickly mold. If you choose not to roast or dehydrate the seeds, they must be refrigerated and used within a few days.

ROASTING SUNFLOWER SEEDS (OPTIONAL):

Roast approximately 15 to 20 minutes at 225 degrees F., or dehydrate at 110 to 115 degrees F. for up to 24 hours.

Because sunflower milk has a tendency to oxidize quickly and turn brown, I recommend that you prepare the milk in small batches and use immediately.

Simple Sunflower Milk
24 ounces

- 3 cups filtered water
- 1 cup sunflower seeds

Blend well.
Strain.

Creamy Sunflower Milk
16 ounces

- 2 cups filtered water
- ½ cup sunflower seeds
- 2 Tablespoons tocotrienols
- 2 teaspoons lecithin

Blend sunflower seeds and water.
Strain.
Pour milk back into a clean blender.
Add tocos and lecithin.
Blend well.

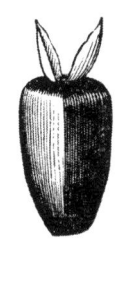

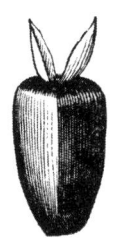

Sweetened Sunflower Milk
16 ounces

- 2 cups filtered water
- ½ cup sunflower seeds
- 2 medjool dates, medium/large, pitted
- 2 Tablespoons tocotrienols
- 2 teaspoons lecithin

Blend the water, sunflower seeds and dates.
Strain the mixture.
Pour the milk back into a clean blender.
Add tocos and lecithin.
Blend well.

Toffee Sunflower Milk
16 ounces

- 2 cups filtered water
- ½ cup sunflower seeds
- 1 medjool date, medium/large, pitted
- 2 Tablespoons tocotrienols
- 2 teaspoons lecithin
- 6 drops toffee flavored stevia*
- ¼ teaspoon vanilla extract

Blend the water, sunflower seeds and date.
Strain the mixture.
Pour milk back into a clean blender.
Add tocos, lecithin, vanilla and flavored stevia.
Blend well.

*Rum stevia extract will also work for this recipe.

Visit our website at www.MilksAlive.com for links to find flavored stevia blends.

Sunflower Banana Milk
16 ounces

- 2 cups sunflower seed milk, simple or creamy
- ¾ cup banana, fresh or frozen
- 2 teaspoons raw honey

Blend well.

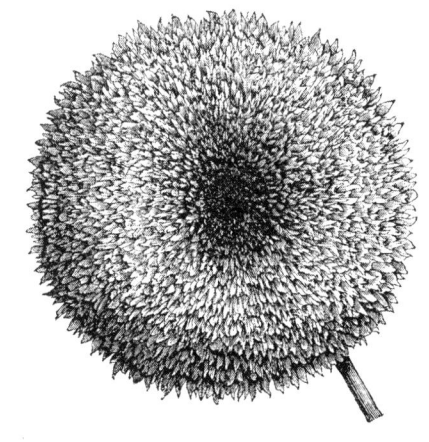

Sunflower Persimmon Cranberry Smoothie

8 ounces

This recipe has delicious cranberry bits in your smoothie!

- 1 cup sunflower seed milk, simple or creamy
- ½ cup ripe persimmon
- 2 Tablespoons unsweetened, dried cranberries
- 1 teaspoon light agave

Blend well, making sure to break up the persimmon and dried cranberries.

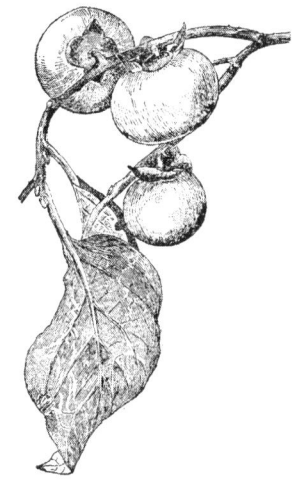

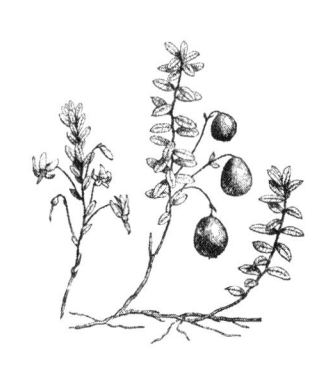

Sunflower Pecan Vanilla Milk

Single 8 ounce serving

- 1 cup filtered water
- ¼ cup sunflower seeds
- 2 Tablespoons pecans
- ⅛ teaspoon stevia
- ⅛ vanilla extract

Blend well.
Strain.

Sunflower Pecan Vanilla Smoothie
Single 8 ounce serving

1	cup filtered water
¼	cup sunflower seeds
2	Tablespoons pecans
½	cup banana, fresh or frozen
2	teaspoons raw honey
⅛	teaspoon vanilla extract

Blend water, sunflower seeds and pecans.
Strain.
Place the milk back into a clean blender.
Add bananas, honey and vanilla.
Blend well.

Sunflower Hemp Grape Coconut Milk
Single 8 ounce serving

1	cup coconut water
¼	cup sunflower seeds
2	Tablespoons hemp seeds
2	Tablespoons unsweetened, organic, frozen grape juice concentrate

Blend all ingredients.
Strain.

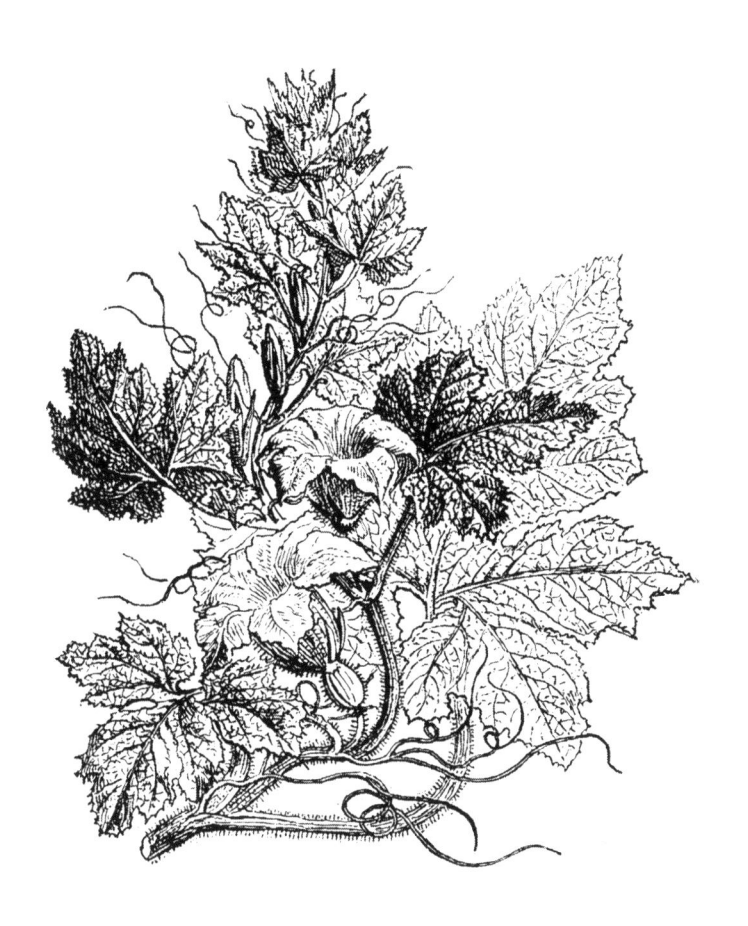

Pumpkin Seed

Pumpkins are native to the Americas and found across north, south and central America. Squashes, corn and beans were three of the earliest domesticated plants in the Western Hemisphere and pumpkin seeds were an important part in many Native Americans diets.

Also known in Spanish as pepita, "little seed of squash," the pumpkin seed is a good source of protein and is high in manganese, magnesium, phosphorus, copper and zinc.

Pumpkin Seed Soak Time:
approximately 10 to 12 hours

If you soak them longer, I recommend rinsing and changing the water about halfway through the process.

Moist, soaked seeds will quickly mold. If you choose not to roast or dehydrate the seeds, they must be refrigerated and used within a few days.

ROASTING PUMPKIN SEEDS (OPTIONAL):

Roast approximately 15 to 20 minutes at 225 degrees F., or dehydrate at 110 to 115 degrees F. for up to 24 hours.

Pumpkin milk has a lovely flavor and is packed with nutrients.

I find that pumpkin milk is best on its own, plain or lightly sweetened and I suggest you use it immediately after preparing.

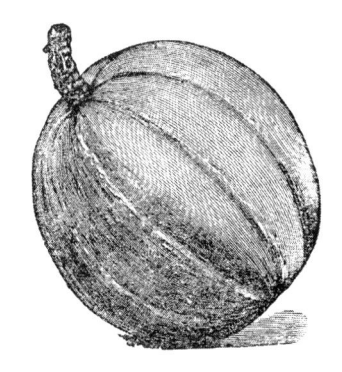

Simple Pumpkin Seed Milk
16 ounces

　　2　cups filtered water
　　½　cup pumpkin seeds

Blend well.
Strain.

Creamy Pumpkin Seed Milk
16 ounces

- 2 cups filtered water
- ½ cup pumpkin seeds
- 2 Tablespoon tocotrienols
- 2 teaspoons lecithin

Blend pumpkin seeds and water.
Strain.
Pour milk back into a clean blender.
Add tocos and lecithin.
Blend well.

Sweetened Pumpkin Seed Milk
16 ounces

- 2 cups filtered water
- ½ cup pumpkin seeds
- 2 medjool dates, medium/large, pitted

Blend well.
Strain.

Pumpkin Seed Wheatgrass Milk
Single 8 ounce serving

- 1 cup filtered water
- ¼ cup pumpkin seeds
- ¼ 4" by 4" container wheatgrass*
- 1 medjool date, medium/large

Blend well.
Strain.

* See Wheatgrass Recipes on page 39.

Creamy Pumpkin Seed Coconut Milk
Single 8 ounce serving

1	cup filtered water
¼	cup pumpkin seeds
1	Tablespoon coconut milk
2	teaspoons coconut palm sugar
1	teaspoon raw honey
2	teaspoons tocotrienols
1	teaspoon lecithin

Blend water and pumpkin seeds.
Strain.
Pour milk back into a clean blender.
Add coconut milk, coconut palm sugar, honey, tocos and lecithin.
Blend well.

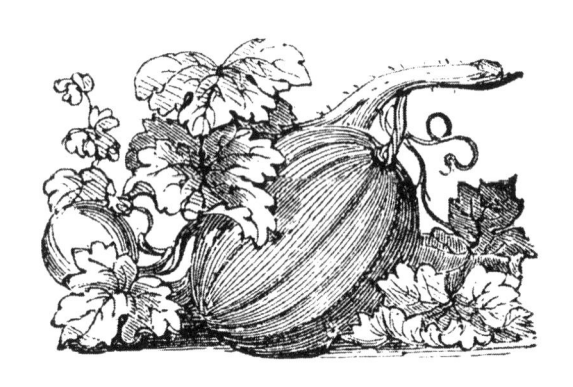

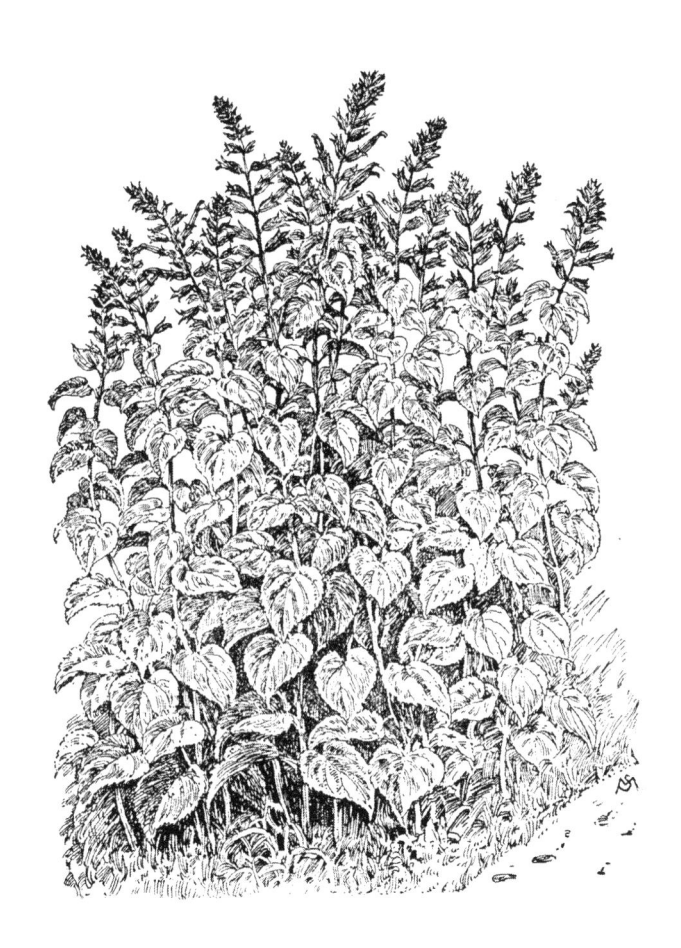

Chia Seeds

Chia, related to the mint family, is a flowering plant that is native to central and southern Mexico and Guatemala. It is believed that the Aztecs cultivated chia in the pre-Columbian era.

Chia is a powerhouse of nutrients and, along with flax and hemp, one of the richest plant sources of Omega 3. These tiny, precious seeds are high in fiber, vitamins, minerals and antioxidants.

Chia, like flax, is a mucilaginous seed. Because of this, you would not make milk from chia in the traditional way of making nut and seed milks. However, the chia seed has an interesting "suspension" property when used with nut milk and iced tea.

Chia seed adds a nutritional punch that does not change the flavor of what you are preparing and adds a great texture. Chia also makes a delicious tapioca-like pudding that does not require cooking.

Chia Seeds with Nut or Seed Milk

The basic ratio is 1 Tablespoon of chia seeds to 8 ounces (1 cup) of liquid. You may prefer more; however, I suggest you try this ratio first.

Prepare your nut or seed milk recipe.
Pour into a mason jar.
Add 1 Tablespoon chia seeds per cup of liquid.
Place the cap on the jar, and shake vigorously.
Refrigerate for a few minutes and shake again.

Repeat this process a few times so the chia stays dispersed and does not clump.

Chia Smoothies

Blending chia seeds adds texture to milk.

The basic ratio is 1 Tablespoon of chia seeds to 8 ounces (1 cup) of liquid. You may prefer more; however, I suggest you try this ratio first.

Prepare your nut or seed milk recipe.
Pour milk back into a clean blender.
Add 1 Tablespoon chia seeds per cup of liquid.
Blend well.

Chia Seed Iced Tea

Chia seed iced tea is excellent with fruity summer teas!

You can find numerous delicious berry, hibiscus and tropical blends at your health food store.

The basic ratio is 1 Tablespoon of chia seeds to 8 ounces (1 cup) of liquid. You may prefer more; however, I suggest you try this ratio first.

Prepare a strong blend of fruity tea.
Sweeten to taste.
Allow tea to cool and pour into a mason jar.
Add 1 Tablespoon chia seeds per cup of liquid.
Place cap on the jar and shake vigorously.
Refrigerate for a few minutes, then shake again.

Repeat this process a few times so the chia stays dispersed and does not clump.

Serve cold with a fruit garnish.

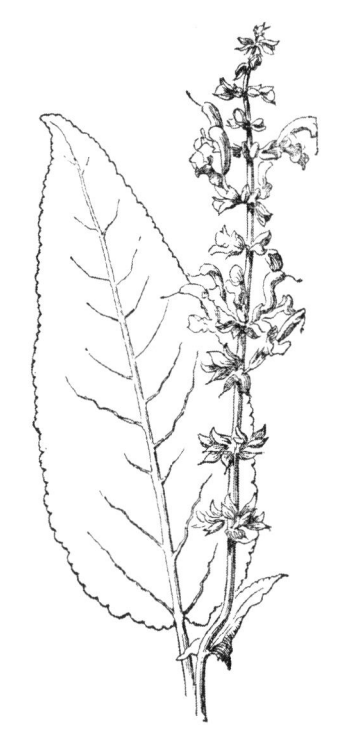

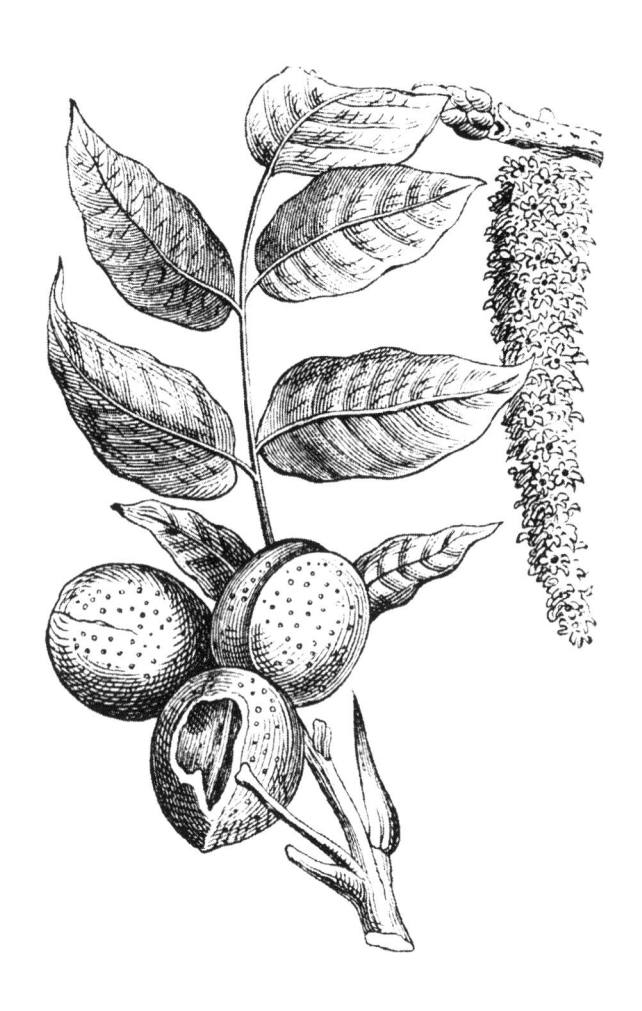

Other Nuts and Seeds

Although, highly nutritious and delicious, I rarely use the nuts and seeds in this chapter for making milk.

I encourage you to include them in your diet, as they add texture and flavor to desserts, savory recipes and smoothies.

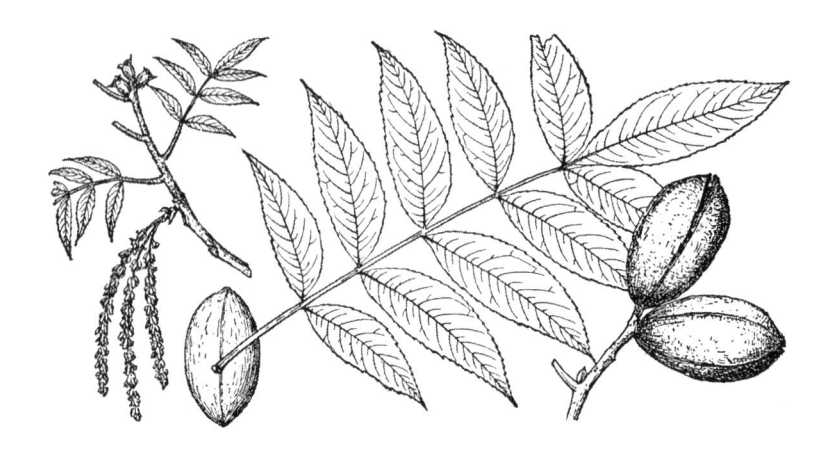

Pecans

The history of pecans has been traced back to the late fifteenth century and pecans are the only major tree nut to grow naturally in North America. Originating in central and eastern North America, wild pecans were prized among the colonial Americans as a delicacy. The name "pecan" is a Native American word of Algonquin origin that was used to describe "all nuts requiring a stone to crack."

Pecans are higher in fat, lower in protein and are an excellent source of vitamins and minerals including vitamins E and A, folic acid, calcium, magnesium, copper, phosphorus, potassium, manganese, several B vitamins and zinc.

Because of the high fat content, keep them refrigerated.

Pecan Soak Time:
approximately 3 hours

Discard soak water.

Pecan Milk

If pecans are one of your favorite nuts, try the following proportion for milk.

- 2 cups filtered water
- ⅔ cups pecans

Blend well.
Strain.
For a sweet pecan milk, add dates or maple syrup.

WAYS TO USE PECANS

PECANS IN DESSERTS

- Pecan pie
- Cookies
- Crusts in raw food preparation
- Added to a trail mix
- Ice creams

PECANS IN SAVORY RECIPES

- Vegan paté
- Roasted
- Savory bread pudding
- Garnish for salads or main courses

Pistachios

Who doesn't love pistachios and the ritual of having to open and enjoy them one nut at a time?

Pistachio trees have grown in the Middle East for thousands of years and in Persia (modern day Iran), pistachio trade and ownership of pistachio groves brought riches and high status. Archeologists have found evidence from excavations in northeastern Iraq that pistachio nuts were a common food as early as 6750 BC.

Today Iran, the United States and Turkey are the major producers of pistachios.

Pistachios contain unsaturated fats and essential fatty acids along with a number of essential vitamins and nutrients and are particularly high in potassium.

WAYS TO USE PISTACHIOS

PISTACHIOS AND DESSERTS

- Baklava
- Biscotti
- Crusts in raw food preparation
- Added to a trail mix
- Ice creams

PISTACHIOS IN SAVORY RECIPES

- Pistachio butter
- Garnishes
- Roasted plain or salted

Pine Nuts

Pine Nuts are the edible seeds of pine cones and are known by many names, including Indian nuts, pinon, pignoli and pignolia. Although called nuts, they are seeds with dozens of varieties from around the world.

Today the Chinese pine nut is often found in the United States because of its availability and price. In the US, pinon nuts come mainly from the Colorado pinon tree, a two-needled pine that grows wild in the states of Colorado, New Mexico, Arizona and Utah.

Pine nuts are a high calorie seed, rich in mono-unsaturated fat. They are an excellent source of vitamin E, B-complex group and contain healthy amounts of essential minerals like manganese, potassium, calcium, iron, magnesium, zinc and selenium.

I love the rich and unique flavor of pine nuts and because they are high in fats and expensive, I don't use them for making milk.

Because of the high fat content, keep them refrigerated.

WAYS TO USE PINE NUTS

PINE NUTS AND DESSERTS

- Cookies
- Cakes

PINE NUTS IN SAVORY RECIPES

- Crackers
- Vegan cheese
- Garnishes for salads and greens
- Garnishes for grain dishes
- Pesto—a combination of walnuts and pine nuts make a great pesto

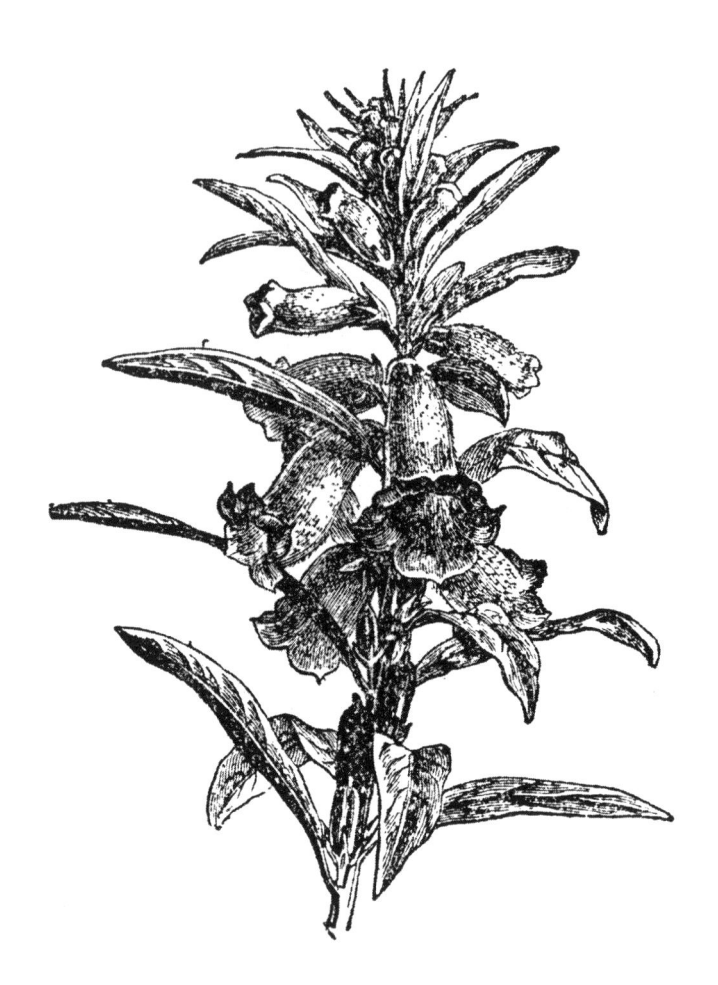

Sesame Seeds

Sesame seeds are used in cuisines around the world and have a rich, nutty flavor. Sesame is considered to be the oldest oil seed crop, domesticated over 5,000 years ago and has the highest oil content of any seed.

Sesame seeds are high in trace minerals and a good source of B complex vitamins and protein.

I love the flavor of sesame seeds and I enjoy the taste of sesame milk and you will find a recipe for peanut and sesame milk in the chapter on peanuts. However, I do find that these seeds are better suited for both desserts and savory recipes.

If sesame is a favorite seed flavor for you, try the following proportion for milk.

Use raw or pan toasted, unsalted sesame seeds.

Sesame Milk

    2   cups filtered water
    1   cup toasted sesame seeds

Blend well.
Strain.
For a sweet sesame milk add honey to taste.

WAYS TO USE SESAME SEEDS

SESAME SEEDS AND DESSERT

- Cookies
- Sesame candy or sesame brittle
- Halvah

SESAME SEEDS IN SAVORY RECIPES

- Crackers
- Breads
- Gomasio: roasted crushed sesame seed with sea salt
- Tahini: makes a delicious spread with miso
- Base for savory sauces, excellent on grains and vegetables
- Garnishes from soups to desserts

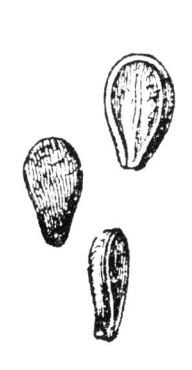

Flax

Flax, also known as linseed, is a widely cultivated plant originally believed to be from the Mediterranean region of Europe. Linseed oil is made from the seeds and the textile, linen, is produced from the stems of the plant.

Flax is a powerhouse of nutrients. Flax seeds are low in carbohydrates yet high in fiber, antioxidants, Omega 3 fatty acids, phytochemicals and vitamins.

Because flax is a mucilaginous seed, I do not recommend using flax for milk.

Flax can be used whole or ground. I recommend that you grind them in small portions and store what you don't use in the refrigerator.

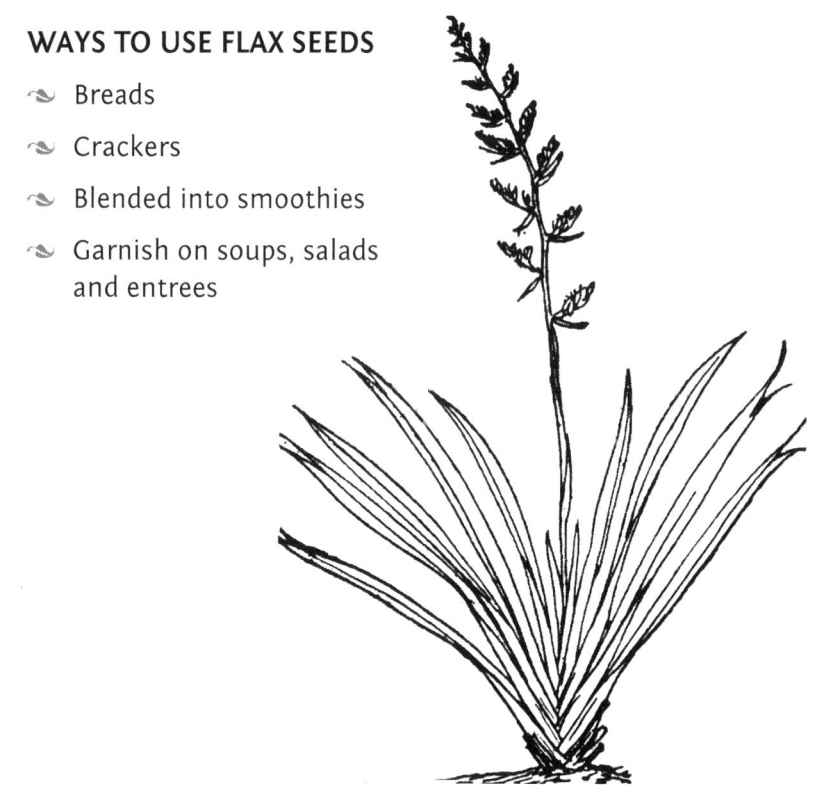

WAYS TO USE FLAX SEEDS

- Breads
- Crackers
- Blended into smoothies
- Garnish on soups, salads and entrees

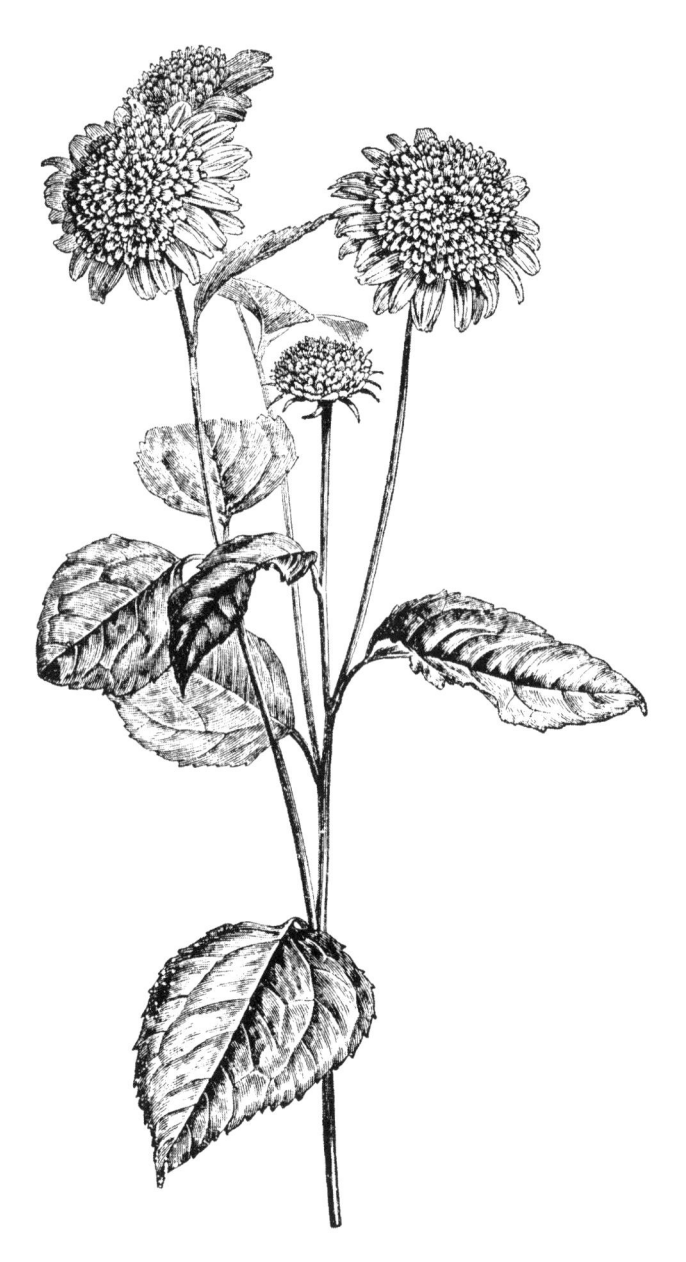

Cheers to re-defining milk!

Visit our website:
www.MilksAlive.com

Printed in Great Britain
by Amazon